The Other Side of the Bed— A Nurse's True Story

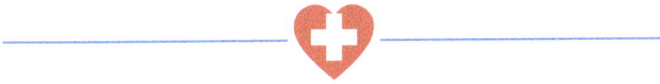

By Georgia Murawski R.N., B.S.N.

Executive Editing and Story Development: Angelica Harris Inc.

Editor: Deanna Ryan-Meister

Design: MeisterWorks Graphic Design
meisterworks.myportfolio.com

All photos by Georgia Murawski and family members
unless otherwise indicated.

Published by Georgia Murawski

Printed by IngramSpark

ISBN: 978-0-578-84001-7

Contents

Dedication

For My Fellow Nurses and Patients Before and During the COVID-19 Crisis, This Book is for You

A S I WRITE THIS, we are in a coronavirus pandemic. I am a nurse, and I have recently been a patient. I was fortunate enough to have had my second abdominal hernia surgery just before the pandemic, and the call for social distancing and isolation. All elective cases were postponed, and many office visits and appointments were cancelled.

Because of the nature of my surgery, I had to go to a doctor's office post-op for the doctor to remove one of the drains. The hospital was a scary scene due to COVID-19. Staff walked the hallways wearing masks and gloves. I was greeted and screened by a nurse who would ask me a few questions at the information desk. Hopefully by the time this book is published, it will be a happier and healthier world out there.

Dr. Anthony Fauci, the federal government's top infectious disease expert, told lawmakers that the novel coronavirus spreading across the globe is 10 times more lethal than the seasonal flu. The flu has a mortality rate of 0.1 percent. The coronavirus has a rate of 10 times that amount. He stated, "That is why we have to stay ahead of the game in preventing this."

It is sad and pathetic to be ill and hospitalized, and to feel alone when you are suffering during COVID. My heart goes out to you.

—Georgia Murawski R.N., B.S.N.

I will now take you through my experiences *on the other side of the bed*. I find it so very crucial to explain this to you. It is my wish that, if you are a patient one day, my story will help make your experience much easier for you to handle. Throughout this book, I will share little tips and guides for you to consider, and to take with you along your journey.

I am with you; You are not alone!

Come and walk the hospital floors with me.

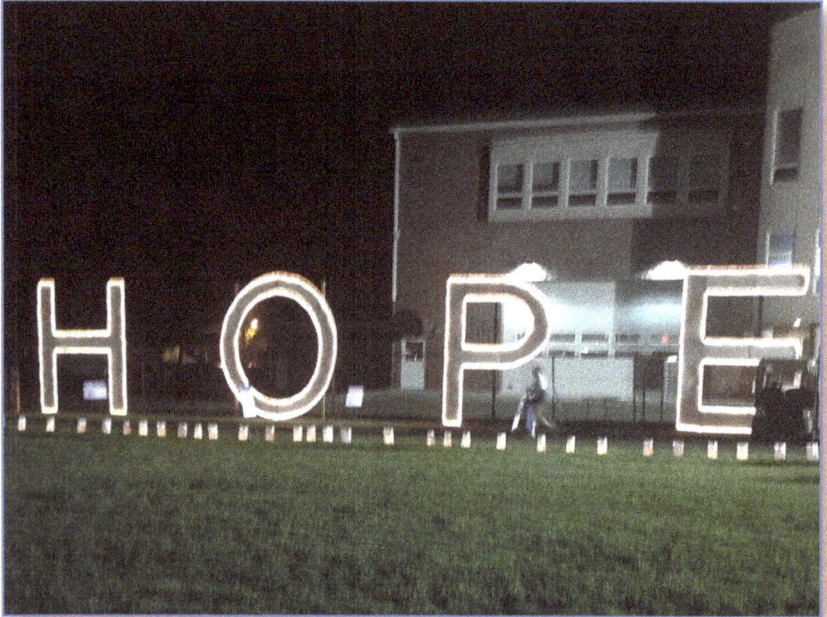

Never Lose Hope. *This photo was taken by me at a breast cancer fundraiser in NY.*

Acknowledgments

HAVING AN IDEA AND THEN to write a book is truly both a hard and surreal process. However, it is ultimately one of the most rewarding journeys I have ever imagined or committed myself to. In celebration of completing this, the following people need to be recognized and be aware of my heartfelt appreciation.

To my parents—I have the utmost gratitude to my awesome mom and dad for bringing me into this fine world. Even though a doctor once told my mom she would "never" have children, she made the impossible a reality. You both worked hard, sacrificed and were dedicated in raising your children.

Mom—For the positive advice and love you shared throughout my hurdles and in my life. When I recently asked you how you deal with sick children, you simply stated, you learn to deal with it and have faith. I will never ever forget when, at age 83, you came on a train from another state with my sister to see me after my major surgery. Even in my groggy state, I saw you quite clearly, and your presence was most comforting.

Dad—When I called out to you from heaven and asked for more strength, I felt your presence with signs from above.

Don—Thank you so very much my dear husband, who endlessly helped me through thick and thin. You kept me afloat and kept me from drowning in many situations. Even my daughter remarked how dad really kept it together at that time. Even being my private driver and being so pleasant about it, will be forever etched in my memory. I wish to express my deepest appreciation for your unstoppable assistance throughout my ordeals.

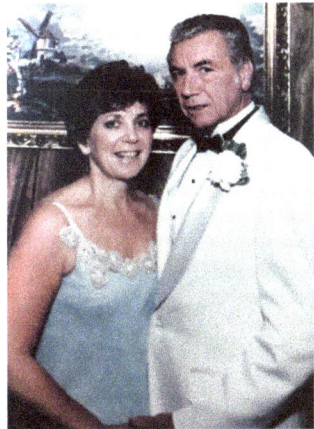

The best parents anyone could ask for!

To my dear children Ryan and Jill who ultimately gave me my title of "mom" and for your praise and well wishes with this book. I clearly remember when one night I sent Jill some paragraphs from my initial writings and she said, "Mom, you are a good writer".

For my siblings:

Cathy—You always went out of your way to help me and I would call you "Johnny on the spot". I could count on you to be positive yet honest. You always got the job done. You are truly a great co-captain. You helped me in many rough situations and I am truly blessed to have you as my sister.

Nancy—Your famous and witty line, "You are in it to win it!" will resonate with me always. I hope to pass this on to someone who may need to hear it. You were always looking for ideas to help me with my pain etc.

Patrick—My only and dynamic brother who would call me and talk to me before and after my surgeries. Your jokes, when I needed to hear them, would lighten the load. I will never forget when I said, "I have God on my right and dad on my left watching me", and you said, "And you have us in the middle". This brought the true essence of family to light.

Karin—My baby sister who is so much like myself; we are bookends. One of my many gifts I received in life came from you— a lovely and very practical journal, that truly inspired me to begin drafting my book. Your steadfast love and respect for your oldest sister is very much cherished by me, now and forever.

To my editors Angelica, Carol and Dee, and to my graphic designer and publishing consultant Neil—you all really helped me get the book started and prepared, and I am truly thankful. You were a pleasure to work with.

Most of all, I must thank very much Our Dear Lord, because without Him I would not be here today. I am vertical and alive because of you, God. The scriptures include a simple phrase, Look back and thank Him, look forward and trust Him. That simple but powerful message is etched in my mind now, and always.

Introduction

I HAD BEEN PUTTING OFF writing this book for many years, although it was on my bucket list for quite some time. Along the way not only have I been a patient, but also a professional nurse with many experiences. I have been sick, and experienced the need of care from my fellow nurses. Those experiences have been priceless. I decided that it was a must to jot down some notes and start writing this book for you from both a nurse's and patient's perspective. I will explain my encounters and guide you, with tips and advice to help direct you as a patient.

The Other Side of the Bed focuses on various separate stories of a nurse and the role reversal of her professional field on numerous instances. To embark on real-life fear, challenges, and the quest of the unknown from one who has truly had ups and downs as a patient. It is my hope to bring to you my experiences through the deep human elements in life's roughest and scariest moments, and how we decide to handle them. As a patient, and even being a nurse, it was that way I accepted and identified my own health issues that I sought out professionals who would help me along many of my life's bumpy moments.

I have been a registered nurse along with receiving my baccalaureate degree for over thirty-four years. Until you have been a patient at some point, you truly do not know what it feels like to be one. I do fully understand, and I totally empathize with you. Being *on the other side as a patient*, is quite different in numerous ways.

With the latest computer technology, nursing has changed dramatically over the years. There is so much clicking and charting that sometimes I feel we miss the hands-on association with the patient. Sometimes I found myself looking at the computer more than the patient. It is our go-to as far as information, but I felt that when using such devices I did not give enough eye-to-eye contact to patients. I would try to do my best to stop what I was doing and chat with the patient. What I found was that eye-to-eye contact and the chat with the patient were key elements in finding out what was really going on. Technology gives us the deep roots into the patient's body and health issues within the nanostructure of its artificial intelligence. But eye-to-eye contact tells us as nurses and doctors the humanity within the illness we are treating. Additionally, attentive listening allows for better diagnostic assessment of the patient's concerns and demonstrates nonverbal respect. Listen carefully, avoid interrupting, and pay close attention to emotional clues. (Laura Cooley catalyst.nejm.org Fostering Human Connection in the Covid 19 NCBI_NIH www.nebi.nlm.nih.gov/pmc articles PMC7371327 May 20, 2020)

When I first started to chart in my early years as a nurse, we had a pen, and pink progress notes. I felt it was a lot quicker than using technology. Imagine that there was no computer charting, and when I wrote the notes down, it helped me to connect more with my patient than that of the computers of today. There was no down time or worrying about whether the computer would go down.

I am truly happy with my career path that I have chosen. Initially, I was a postpartum nurse; I worked with mothers who had just given birth in the labor and delivery department. Wanting more of a challenge, I was intrigued by the operating room and wanted to see if that was truly my area of passion. I proceeded to venture into the main operating room. Boy was that a quest of learning! I rotated to the various units for about six weeks learning the different specialties, including plastic surgery, orthopedic, (musculoskeletal), general surgery, urology, (urinary system) burn, heart, and ophthalmology (eyes). Once I rotated through all the units, I made my way to ambulatory surgery, that was my greatest joy. I learned many new and exciting things about the world in the operating room. I was thrilled that I switched over to learn about this new horizon. Looking back on my career, it gave me my greatest adventures working in the operating room and performing with many special and skilled individuals who shared the same interest and love for their job.

As years went by and I had my dear children, Ryan, and Jillian, I would teach classes on baby care to moms- and dads-to-be to prepare for the birth of their child. It was both very satisfying and rewarding in many ways. It was fascinating to see the attentiveness of these individuals during the class. There were many tips, guides, handouts, and videos to show them how to make the journey a bit easier when their baby or babies arrived. Also, there was much less charting to do. I did love that aspect of nursing towards the end of my career, along with going back to postpartum floor duty.

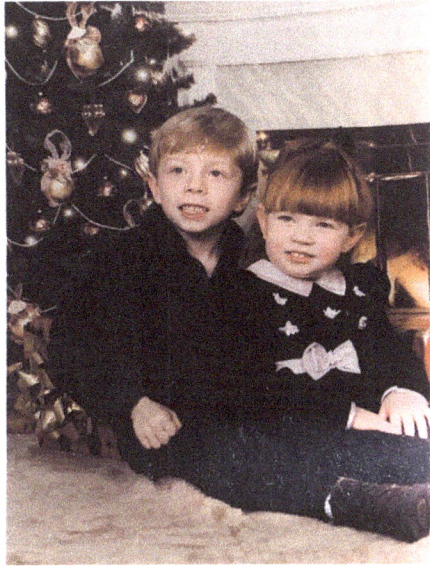

One of my greatest joys and accomplishments. (Photo was taken by a professional photographer.)

Now, as a retired nurse, who has been a patient, medicine has changed dramatically, both in normal times and with the onset of COVID-19. Within these pages are written my journal entries of the good and the bad of medicine.

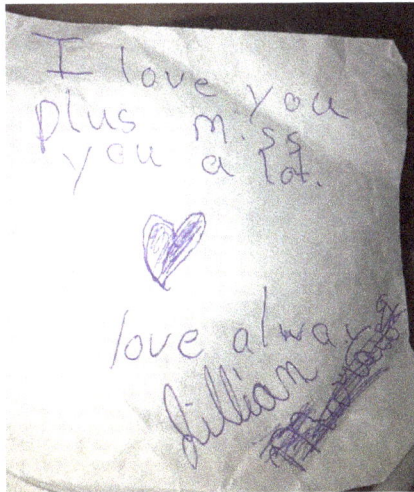

One of many treasured handmade notes from Jill.

"The human element of an in-person health care encounter cannot fully be replaced by a virtual one. After all, a provider's gentle but appropriate touch can sometimes convey empathy in a way that words cannot. However, identifying and improving one's skills for engaging in meaningful virtual communications with patients and colleagues can help ensure that human connection prospers in the midst of, and beyond, the changes brought by the COVID-19 pandemic."

— Laura Cooley PhD Senior Director, Education and Outreach, Academy of Communication in Healthcare
Nashville, Tennessee 5/20/2020

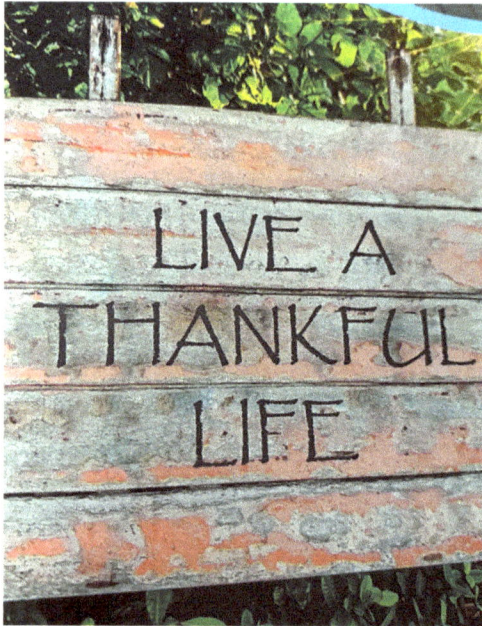

Doctor's Visits or Follow Ups

WE HAVE ALL BEEN TO a doctor's office at some point in our lives. Isn't it funny how we make an appointment but rarely see the doctor at the time scheduled? Be prepared to wait a half hour to an hour later, or at times longer, before you are called-in after registering. I usually bring a sweater, and a book or magazine, or play games on my phone to pass the time.

What I find significant to do is to make a list of questions you may want to ask your doctor. I never care how many questions I must ask. I'd rather inquire and get my answers than to leave for home, and say, "Why did I not seek out my concerns?" I still make my list to this day whenever I see a doctor. Doctors are genuinely happy to answer any concerns you may have for them. A doctor once told me that the patients just do not ask questions. There are no silly or dumb inquiries.

If you are wondering what to ask, here are some sample suggestions: *What do you think is ailing me? Can it be treated with medications or will I need surgery? Do you have an initial diagnosis?* If the doctor recommends medication first, then ask, *What other symptoms will I see? Is it hereditary and treatable? Is there anything else I should look for? Are there side effects to the medications?*

This is a good time to make sure all the medications you have been taking are up-to-date and determine if any refills are needed. You may be asked to provide a list of your medications. You can bring them or have the names written down or entered in your phone. Make sure you take your meds completely and do not skip any as prescribed by your doctor, even if you feel better. Follow the prescription as stated on the bottle and as per physician order.

For example, blood pressure medication is more effective when taken at night. What time of day a patient takes blood pressure medication can have an impact on its effectiveness. According to Dr. Howard Lewine, taking blood pressure pills at night might improve blood pressure and prevent heart attacks and/or strokes. (Eur Heart J. Oct 22, 2019)

However, there is a crucial question to always ask the doctor: May the new prescription interact with another medication you are currently taking? It could cause a bad allergic reaction or can counteract (go against) one of your medications and cancel it out altogether. This can be dangerous. Many times, the pharmacist will know best regarding medications and interactions. Finally, before you leave, ask for a doctor's note if you may need one when returning to work, school etc.

If a doctor prescribes a medication, ask the office staff if they have any samples. It helps not only with the cost, but it gives you a trial of the medicine you are about to use. I once asked if the office manager if she had a medication that includes an active ingredient famotidine,which helps to relieve heartburn. It does this by reducing the amount of acid in the stomach. I have asked and it worked out well. A doctor ordered me to take the pills for 14 days and she gave me a 14-day supply. There may be times, however, that your prescription will be longer in duration. Your insurance may cover more long-term use of a particular medication. Keep in mind that you can ask for a ninety-day mail order supply, as it is cheaper and it is conveniently mailed to you. Also, see if you can be prescribed a generic brand that may work just as well and be cost-effective.

Personally, as a patient, I try my best to become friendly with the staff members. If they do not have an identification tag, ask them their name. I put it in my phone near my doctor's office number. This way, I can associate a name and a face. It becomes a more familiar thing. When I worked in the hospital, I loved when patients remembered my name. I learned along the way that it is a sweet gesture to bring in small goodies for the staff especially if you will have repeated visits in the future. This is most appreciated and sometimes when they are busy a great snack always helps if they have not had lunch or a recent break. When I was a nurse, and a patient would bring to our nurses station a tray of cookies or a basket of fruit, we were very appreciative—at times that cookie or apple was the only thing we ate on our 12-hour shift.

Another iota for any patient who is under a doctor's care, is to find out if they were going to be "on call" which means the doctor is on duty over the next weekend. This way I always felt that if I need him or her, I knew they were just a phone call away. As a patient, it made me feel extremely secure. They usually respond quickly if you call the office.

Dermatology is another form of medicine. It addresses diseases of the skin, from acne to dermatitis, to moles, or something you need to have removed. Procedures can be easily done right in their office setting, or they may schedule you for another appointment and perform local anesthesia to the area they need to excise if it is small and easy for them. However, moles can be cancerous—if your doctor tells you to remove it, do so right away, before it escalates and you have a serious issue on your hands. Remember local anesthesia wears off in a couple of hours unless they use a longer-acting medicine. They will give you instructions to care for your wound and pain medications. Note to self, you may have to come back for a follow-up visit. Always follow up—it is vital for your healing and overall wellness. Skin cancer is on the rise. There are three types of skin cancer: basal, squamous and melanoma. I do have a fair amount of skin cancer history with my immediate family, and we must be checked vigilantly to help prevent skin cancer or to catch it in its early stages.

One time when I was a teenager, I had to get three cysts, called chalazions, removed from my eyelids. My mom brought me to a Manhattan hospital that specializes in eyes ears nose and mouth. It is much like an operating room, where you have a day procedure and after recovery. I remember that a small-framed resident approached my bedside and told me what to expect during the surgery and after. Although we did not know much at the time,

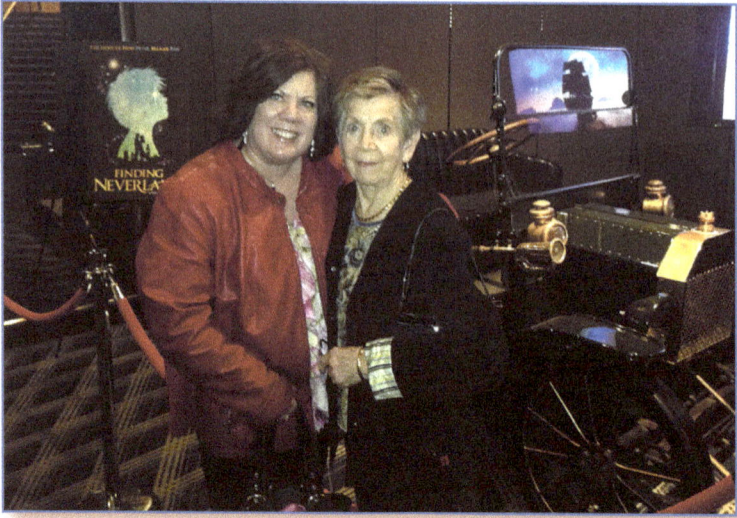

My Mom~My Lifeline

my mom assured me that all would be alright, and I felt better about it. My dad wanted to be with me but had to wait in the car due to the craziness of parking in Manhattan.

The physician put local anesthesia directly into my upper and lower eyelids. I could feel the fluid run down my face and had to sit real still to get the cysts removed. I remember him telling me he had to wait a few minutes for my eyes to feel numb before he proceeded. I was so happy once the cysts were removed. They truly were an eyesore—so to speak—in more ways than one.

Another situation was when I had a growth on the left side of my neck. It looked as though I had swallowed a golf ball. I had to have general anesthesia and surgery to have it removed. What I did not know at that time was the difference between benign (not harmful in effect) and malignant (invasive) in cases of cancer. I am sure it caused a lot of stress on my parents, as they were worried that their daughter may indeed have cancer. When we were told it was a benign cyst, my parents and I were very much relieved. After dealing with eye and throat lumps, I have concluded that I am very cystic.

Have you ever had a mammography? According to an article in *Radiology*, "Mammography is specialized medical imaging that uses a low-dose x-ray system to see inside the breasts. A mammography exam, called a mammogram, aids in the early detection and diagnosis of breast diseases in women." (www.radiologyinfo.org) "With mammography you want to get an accurate one with high quality images and a good reading of that image (Susan G. Komen). The American College of Radiology states, "One out of every six diagnoses of breast cancer occur in women 40-45, and three out of four women diagnosed with cancer have no family history and are not considered high risk."

I anticipate that if you are a female, at some point you will have, or have had a mammogram. All I can say is that the intense pressure of the procedure is like having a vice squeezing on your breast tissue. The one consolation is the quickness of this test. If you have an exceptionally good technician, it will be done promptly. It is unnerving to see the other women waiting for their imaging tests, and to wait after your test for the technician to ensure the readings were clear and not have to be repeated. Afterward, waiting for the results can be a bit nerve-wracking, whether you receive either positive or negative results. Make sure to consistently have a mammogram done as instructed by your doctor. Don't fall behind.

As a nurse, I recommend that you do a self-check of your breasts once a month, or right after your period, to detect any lumps or changes. By doing this you can save your own life, because early detection is the best detection of all. If you feel something, call your doctor. Remember, not everything that you feel may be cancer.

CAT Scans and MRI Tests

CAT SCAN OR CT SCAN, is an x-ray image using a form of tomography in which a computer controls the motion of the x-ray source and detectors and therefore processes the data and in turn produces an image CT scans show a tumor's shape, size and location. They can even show blood vessels that feed the tumor. By comparing CT scans, they can see if the tumors are shrinking or responding to a treatment or find out if a cancer has come back. To help them see images even more clearly, you may need a special dye called a contrast media. The contrast media helps to improve the radiologist's ability to review the images inside the body (hopkins-medicine.org). It is done to specifically to diagnose muscle and bone disorders such as bone tumors or fractures; pinpoint a location of a tumor, infection, or blood clot; and detect internal bleeding and or injuries (Mayo Clinic).

During a CT scan, you are briefly exposed to ionizing radiation. It is greater than an x-ray, but it gathers more information. If you are getting the contrast dye, you will either take it orally beforehand or have an intravenous line put in and have it given through the intravenous. If you have any blood work done, it must be done before the dye contrast is given, otherwise it will alter the results of your blood work. It may cause an allergic reaction or cause a stomach upset. Notify your doctor as soon as possible if this occurs.

I have had quite a few CT scans with and without dye. They may tell you to take an oral form of dye to drink with instructions before you get it done. I did not do well with the oral version, as it made my stomach quite sick. I called the office and told my doctor what I experienced. I cannot tolerate the oral form. From that point on, it was decided that I will be given intravenous dye with this test. I prefer this route of delivery, as it is quick, and I do not have to taste it.

A Magnetic Resonance Imaging scan (MRI) is a common procedure around the world (Medical News Today Newsletter).

It is a non-invasive and painless procedure, created by Raymond Damadian. He nicknamed the full body scan *The Indomitable*.

MRI machines are long tubular Artificial Intelligence Robots that allow the radiologist to see the inside of every part of your body. The scanner itself typically resembles a large tube with a table in the middle allowing the patient to slide in. It differs from a CT scan and x-rays as it does not have potentially harmful ionizing radiation. It can detect anomalies of the brain and spine, tumors, breast cancer or injuries to the joints, certain types of heart conditions and evaluation of pelvic pain in women.

During the scan, it is vital to stay very still; any movement can disrupt the images. At times, it may be required of you to hold your breath and the technician will talk with you via an intercom. They can hear you and you can hear them.

MRI machines can be very confining. It is tight quarters and it can be even more scary if you are afraid of closed-in spaces. If you are afraid of closed, confined spaces, perhaps you can be assigned an open-sided imaging machine. You may have to wait a bit longer to have it scheduled if they do not have many open-ended units.

When I had the CAT scan done, a genuinely nice, middle-aged employee who was dressed in casual attire was highly informative. He told me what I would be expecting as far as sensations. I was so glad he did because it helped me understand these were normal happenings. The sensations were a warm feeling starting at the neck area that worked itself down to the chest area. It continued to move down and after the chest area I did not feel anything. It came on quickly, then dissipated.

It is also important that you have the prescription (script) for the test. Keep it in your wallet to show them what test you are having if it is an outpatient test. If you forget your script, they can call the office that it was ordered from and get it faxed over to where you are being tested. The test is not too bad. They keep you warm and give you a pillow for under your head and one for under your knees for extra comfort. The machine can be quite noisy also, with various intermittent banging sounds as well. Do not be frightened of these sounds, as they are a normal part of the scanning process. They usually play music for you to listen to.

Drink plenty of water afterwards to help flush out the dye in the body. I am not actually fond of plain water, so I add fruit; blueberries or an orange to enhance the flavor. It also helps to add some natural sugar to your water just in case you feel light-headed after the test.

Blood Tests

ONCE YOU ARE SEEN BY A DOCTOR, either as an inpatient or outpatient, the doctor may order various lab tests. An inpatient is a person who is formally admitted to a hospital of healthcare setting. An outpatient is a patient who a doctor treats and will receive ambulatory care at a hospital or healthcare unit, but may not spend the night and is not formally admitted in the facility. The doctor will order various labs pertinent to what he/she suspects is ailing you. Sometimes you may be referred for a fasting test, which means nothing to eat or drink at least 8 to 12 hours before your blood is drawn. You may be sent to your local laboratory or have it done where you are. The results typically come back relatively quickly. If you are waiting a while for a call back with notification of results, phone your doctor. Hopefully, in the future, it will be faster to find out the results. I hope the results of any test we may have to take will eliminate the agonizing period of waiting for the results.

Recently, I went to a lab and they did not have my orders for blood in the computer database. The doctor had not provided me with a script either. A young girl on staff, wearing a long, high ponytail continued to look at her computer said, "They are not here in the computer."

I said, "Okay, then please call my doctor's office and ask them to fax it over to you."

The manager, a tall lanky male around forty years old, with a bit of a receding hairline and wearing round dark glasses, got on the phone and said to me,

"I am sorry, the computers are down."

To be honest I was a bit annoyed but as a nurse myself I know what it is like to work in a hospital and be on that side of the station. I just looked at the gentleman and said,

"Okay, I will just sit and wait." He suggested that I come back the next day.

I said, "Oh no, I am waiting." I had been sitting there for about an hour when the office manager came over and said, "Mrs. Murawski, the doctor is not on duty to give the order."

I explained, "Sir, I am a nurse and it should be written in my chart." I started to pick up the phone, "I am calling them right now."

To say the least, my anger was mounting. He walked away and low and behold, he came running to me a minute later with the order flashing in his hand. I was so pleased to have had it done, and when I walked out I said to myself, sometimes persistence does pay off.

There was one time when I had the unique displeasure of having the wrong test taken, although it was correctly written down on the script. The office called and said they did the wrong test, and that I should come back and have it redone. It was my mistake. As a nurse, I should have verified the type of blood test. Yes, I was annoyed at myself, but to anyone who was in my position, it was quite normal to depend on others. I will be more observant and double-check when having testing done in future.

Nurse or doctor, when you are the patient and on the other side of the bed, everything changes, you are now in the seat of the emotional, scared out of your wits patient, and you are in need of the help and support that you would give to your patients in the hospital.

I learned to be more careful with my own needs. I also learned to ask for the normal range. There are parameters for normal ranges for each blood test. When the results are out of the normal range, the area indicated is starred or highlighted and brought to your attention by that signal to indicate abnormal result. These parameters allowed me to determine whether it was close to normal, or on the higher aspect of normal.

Infusions and Intravenous

I HAVE HAD TO GO to an outpatient unit for my diagnosis for low iron deficiency. I had asked my medical specialist, a noticeably short and stocky attending physician, to order additional labs at my office visit. I kept complaining of upper thigh pain, and told him it was so very painful when I would lay down.

He said, "Georgia, all your labs are normal, I will see you in three to four months."

I said, "These thighs hurt, can you order more tests to see what the problem is?" Then I continued, "I can go to my laboratory and get it done."

He said, "Sit right there, I will have someone draw your blood to make sure you are manufacturing enough iron."

A few minutes later the phlebotomist came in and drew a few tubes of blood.

Consequently, the results came back that I had an extremely low iron count. My doctor told me that I would have to go to the hospital infusion unit and undergo treatments of an intravenous infusion for iron deficiency. I have found it helpful, on occasion, when the physician would draw a diagram or picture, that gave me a better understanding and clearer perspective when written on paper.

If you have never had an intravenous before, you will be met by a team of nurses in the outpatient unit who are there to help you in every way they can. Once you have checked in, a nurse will come and put a rubber tourniquet around your arm that helps the nurse find the vein in your arm or hand. The nurse will clean the area, and prick your skin with a small needle attached to a tube. It may hurt going in the vein. Some patients who see the blood fill the vial may get dizzy.

Once the tube is in the vein, they will remove the tourniquet from around your arm and wrap the tube that is inserted in the site, to make sure that it does not fall out during your procedure. As a nurse, I have had to administer these countless times to many patients. I try not to make them uncomfortable. The intravenous should only hurt for a few minutes after input. If it does hurt, tell the nurse immediately. If the area looks swollen or red at the site, the nurse could apply a warm compress, and maybe give you some Tylenol®.

The infusion units are usually facilitated by multiple nurses. It was due to these good and compassionate nurses that for the most part my treatments, scripted for one week apart, were a good experience. You sit in a recliner and they start an intravenous and give you a pillow and blanket to make you are more comfortable. If these are not offered to you, just ask. They will provide what was ordered by your doctor, as this is what you need to help you improve the quality of your health.

IV Centers in hospitals are usually nicely decorated to give you a positive environment, especially due to patients having immune therapy or chemotherapy, etc. Immune therapy uses substances to stimulate or suppress the immune system to help the body fight cancer, infections or other diseases. One thing I do know is that I will need more blood work in the future, and may have to submit to more infusions. If it is for my own good, I am fine with that.

During your treatments, your vital signs are monitored before, during, and after it is completed. Once the nurse comes in and the tube is extracted, the nurse will apply pressure to the open vein to stop it from bleeding, then bandage it. They will also ask you to remain in your seat for at least thirty minutes before you leave to see if you are feeling any dizziness or side-affects. You may also eat and drink or if you wish, sleep while getting this treatment done. Many times, you are permitted to have someone with you, so that if you are not feeling well after your treatment, someone can drive you home.

Years ago, my son Ryan needed to fast and get blood work. As he looked at the site where they were drawing blood, he experienced pallor in his face, and looked like he would pass out. Ryan was sitting at the time but as a nurse and a parent, I acted quickly. I put his legs up on my shoulders and asked the nurse for milk or juice. I kept talking to my son and said, "Stay with me". His legs, with his sneakers and thick muscular calves were still up high on my shoulders. The staff was not helpful at all. You would think they were used to incidences like this, and the fact that people get light-headed due to fasting, or at the sight of blood. Ryan came around quickly, and they removed the vials of blood and needle so he would not see them.

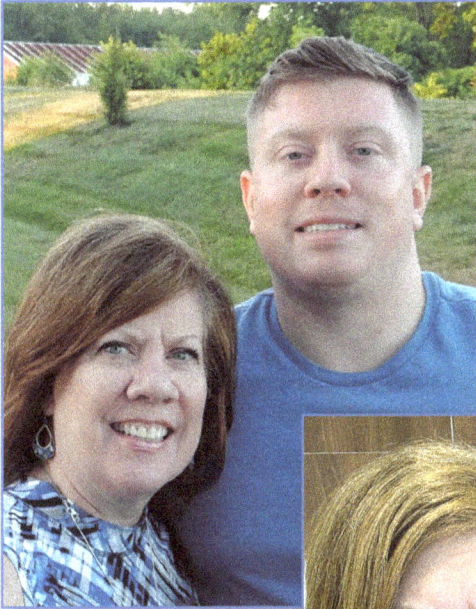

#1 Son!

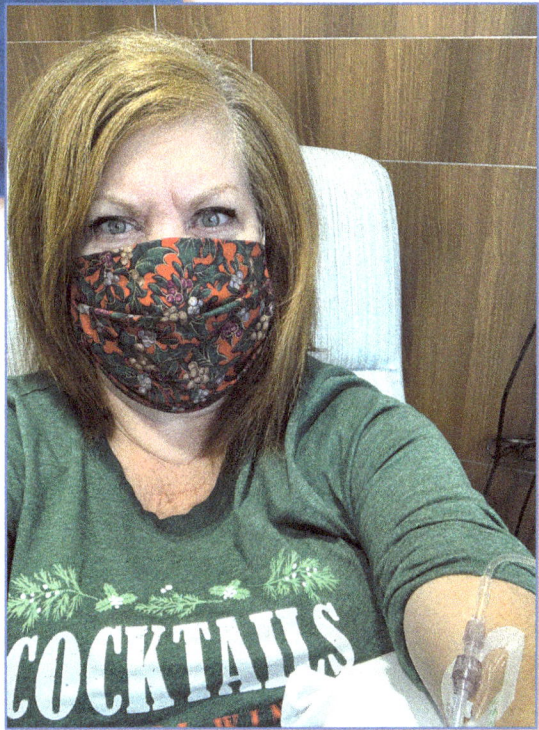

Selfie, day one of a two-day IV iron infusion in an IV infusion center near my house in Delaware.

Endoscopy—
Upper and Lower

A T SOME POINT in time you will need an endoscopy, whether it is an upper or lower scope, that is basically a long hose with a camera connected. It is sent down your throat to check on diseases of the throat and upper stomach.

A colonoscopy is the best protection against colon cancer, the third most common type of cancer in the United States. A colonoscopy allows the doctors to check the colon for polyps and remove them before they become problematic, as polyps can form into cancerous tumors. Like me, some of you will have to have a colonoscopy earlier in your life due to a family history, or early onset cancer. It is quite important to get a baseline test.

Your doctor will give you instructions for the prep to be done the day before the test. He will also give you a prescription for a controlled laxative to help cleanse your bowel. It is specific to each doctor but in essence, it is the same. The day before, you will drink clear liquids, such as ginger ale, apple juice, lemon ices, gelatin, black tea, and coffee. One rule of thumb here, do not eat or drink anything red such as cherry juice or cherry gelatin. The red dye in those food items (if not cleansed properly from the bowel) can look like blood in the bowel during the test.

The night before the test, you will have to drink this horrible tasting drink. Some of you may be required to mix a prescription laxative powder or dissolve a tablet in water. To make it a bit more palatable, try mixing the powder to a mixture of half water and half flat ginger ale. To ensure the ginger ale is flat, let the bottle or can stay open on the kitchen counter until the carbonation is gone. No matter which prep you choose, if you drink it with a straw, it will allow the liquid to bypass most of your taste buds. Make sure it is cold. The prep is worse than the procedure itself. I held my nose while drinking it. If you are lucky enough, you may be given a pill form, but there are certain criteria you must meet to get it.

The prep will certainly cleanse you which, frankly, is not a bad thing. You will go to the bathroom (as my neighbor calls it, 'the throne') most frequently. Get the softest toilet paper and perhaps some baby wipes.

On the day of the procedure, you may wake up with an appetite and want to eat whatever is in front of you, or the thought of food may make you nauseous. Once you get to the ambulatory unit and check in, the nurse will ask you to confirm that you have not eaten or drank anything since the night before. The nurse will do your vitals, start an intravenous, and administer a short acting anesthetic so you will have a nice sleep.

During the colonoscopy, while the colonoscope (a camera attached to the end of a tube) is scanning your colon for anything abnormal such as ulcers or lesions, the camera may show your doctor that you may have polyps. If you do, they will biopsy them and you must wait a few days for the results.

Remember, never take aspirin or any anti-inflammatory before or after your test. If a biopsy was performed, aspirin or prescription blood thinners such as Coumadin can thin the blood and make you bleed. If you do not have any polyps, you may have to see the doctor in a few years or so depending on your doctor's advice. Once the test is done, you may be given some tea and crackers to help with your low blood sugar, and if you are feeling well enough you will be released to go home. You must also have someone drive you home. You cannot drive for 24 hours as the anesthesia remains in your system for a few days and may impair your concentration while driving. Relax as much as possible that day, as you may feel sleepy. Drink water, and eat in slower increments.

Pain Scale

WE ALL EXHIBIT PAIN in different ways. I used to have a high tolerance for it, but after all the illnesses and surgeries, my body has changed drastically. There are times when pain becomes intolerable. If it reaches a point where you have taken pain medications up to the highest dosage and you no longer can handle it, get to an emergency room or urgent care. Once you arrive tell the receptionist immediately that you are in such pain you cannot wait to be seen. When you are in the examining room in your physicians' office or in triage, the doctor or Physician's Assistant will usually ask you to tell them, on a scale of 1 to 10, your pain number based on your level of pain. The higher the number, the more pain is experienced. It is hard to judge, and the pain may not allow you to think clearly. They now have these emojis on the wall where you can point to the face of the emoji that best describes your pain levels.

Once I was in enough agony that I said my pain was an 11—that is how intense my torment was at that time. All pain is individual, but it can frankly knock you for a loop and exhaust you. It can make you cranky or irritable; it can also make you delirious. It could make you scream, or make you not want to talk. I have cried on numerous occasions from suffering. Some people have fainted when in intense pain. There were many times I thought I would lose my mind and felt like giving up. You think it will never end.

Heat and cold therapy are often recommended to help relieve aching muscle or joint pain. Cold helps to reduce swelling. Heat increases the blood flow to an area, and can also relax tight and sore muscles. In some cases, alternating heat and cold may help to increase blood flow to the injury site.

For cold therapy, an ice pack is recommended. I have used a bag of vegetables from the freezer—yes freezer—as an ice pack, as it is both flexible and very convenient. For heat therapy, a re-heatable bean bag, hot water bottle, or heating pad is useful to alleviate muscular pain. I bought a handmade bean bag a few years back, and have used it on numerous occasions to ease my discomfort. You can also apply wet heat by placing a damp hand towel in the microwave for about a minute, depending on the wattage of your microwave. Make sure the damp towel is not too hot when you place it on the pain site.

I have learned that simply applying Vicks® VapoRub™as a topical analgesic can help as well. Its warming agents and herbal extracts include camphor, menthol, and Eucalyptus oil. Eucalyptus oil has antibacterial, antiviral, and anti-inflammatory properties that may help soothe pain and reduce swelling. (Cited: Oct 16, 2019)

You can also treat pain with over-the-counter medication that you may have in your house, or a prescription given by your doctor. If it is a narcotic, a doctor will either write a prescription for you to bring to your pharmacy or send it in online to your pharmacist. It is mandated they see the actual copy. It is essential to write down when you take the medications and how much because as I know, you may not remember when you took one last. Medications do have a maximum amount to be taken in a 24-hour period. Physicians are cautious not to prescribe too many narcotics due to the risk of dependency, as some pain medications called Opioids are addictive substances. I also keep handy the medication list provided by the pharmacy, that includes symptoms and things to look for. To be honest here, thank God I am a nurse, because I must admit that I do refer to a pharmacological book that lists drugs and their side effects. For the lay-person who does not have the book, you can Google the side effects, ask a pharmacist, or ask for the medication list that will have them listed. This way, if you have an unusual symptom, you can see if it is normal to experience. Please be aware of any expired medications you may have by checking on the box or container for the expiration date. Expired drugs can make you extremely sick or can be deadly.

A sitz bath is another form of comfort if you have pain. It is a shallow bath that cleanses the perineum, which is the space between the rectum and either the vulva or scrotum. It is usually effective, and can provide relief from pain, soreness, or itching. The water has to be very warm but tolerable before submersion It is recommended to sit on it for at least 20 minutes and at least twice a day.

I highly recommend this, having used it on several occasions as a patient, with excellent relief of discomfort that I was experiencing. The warm water and sitz bath helps you feel so much better. As a nurse, I have explained to mothers who had just given birth how to use it.

Another device is a shower wand that you can remove from the showerhead. It works well at cleansing areas you may not be able to reach. It is a wide showerhead and the wand can be removed from the stand. It provides warmth and comfort as well. I am not trying to persuade you or make you buy it, but it does help. I am glad I had previously bought it. I only used this at home not in the hospital setting.

You may also be given a medicine ball, that provides gravity-staged medicine in the incision site for pain relief. It is called ON~Q pump that has a balloon type pump filled with local anesthesia that reaches the nearby nerve endings. It has a tube that is inserted into the patient via a catheter, and is stitched in place. This is usually given primarily when you have surgery and is ordered by your physician. It stayed in me for seventy-two hours. Gradually over time the balloon pump deflates, and the medication is dispersed to the operative site. As a nurse, I did not use this device or see it. I only encountered it once as a patient. (avanospainmanagement.com/technicalbulletins)

The ball was removed by a physician before I went home after my surgical procedure, by cutting the sutures to remove it. It provided extra relief from my operative discomfort. I was glad I had it because it did reduce my suffering in the operative site. It does not hurt when it is removed.

Emergency Room Visits

TYPICALLY, YOU NEED to go to an emergency room if you have a lot of pain or a deep cut, bad headache, or something that requires immediate care. It is urgent to go to the ER, whether it is by ambulance or having someone drive you. If you are able ahead of time, it may be a good idea to pack an overnight bag; put your glasses, phone, charger, toothbrush, toothpaste, a sweater, beach sandals or slippers to use while walking, and extra underwear in the bag. If they admit you, at least you have some essentials to help make your stay more comfortable. Most importantly, take along your medications in their original prescription bottles. This will give the triage and admissions office a way to log-in your medications, and make sure that the hospital doctors have your current list of prescriptions on their charts. This way, in the event you are admitted, you will be receiving your correct daily medications that are vital to your healing.

Heading to the emergency room can be quite frightening. Try your best to stay calm and cool, especially to family members or to whoever is taking you. If an ambulance has been called, keep your door open for them. Usually when you arrive, many people are waiting to be seen or treated. They will request your insurance cards and a picture of your license if you drive. If you are in the computer system, they may just ask has anything regarding insurance or address changed. I advise you to bring a sweater or jacket because it can get chilly there. I have been to many emergency rooms and each time I prayed for good staff. I also prayed that it would not be too busy, but a good staff was my main priority.

I really appreciated when the staff addressed themselves by name. It became a bit more personal and I loved it when patients would remember me. If they do not tell you their name, just ask them. I feel it puts the patient at ease a bit to associate a name and a face.

Each of the emergency rooms I had gone to over the years varied in some form. Some were terribly busy, dirty hospitals. Some were awfully slow and disorganized, and some were the complete opposite. I felt it was a bonus to have a clean and efficiently-run facility. Those were my two priorities as a patient.

Once you are being treated, you will get an identification band and an allergy band if you have allergies. Once you are in a cubicle, you may or may not be asked to put on a gown and non-skid bootie socks. The stretcher can be raised for added comfort at both the head and at the feet. There are buttons on the side rail. If you are cold, ask for a blanket or pillow. I remember once a nurse brought me a warmed blanket. I was so thrilled; it was a great gesture. It is the little things that matter sometimes. The non-skid socks keep your feet warm and prevent patients from falling or sliding. Sometimes depending on the hospital, the siderails of the bed may have a nurse's call button. Please be aware to keep the call button close by to press if you need staff assistance. Perhaps clip it to the bed or wrap it around the side rail. I have had my call button fall to the floor, and it was quite a challenge to retrieve it.

Depending on your situation, they may start an intravenous. If you are a bit dehydrated, it may be hard to find a vein. Try to keep warm, as it helps with finding a vein. Sometimes if they miss the vein, you can get bruised. It may take a little while for the bruise to go away. This has happened to me, and there were various colors at the IV site before it disappeared.

Oh, the waiting game with seeing a doctor and waiting to be examined, with possible tests to be done. Let them fully explain to you what they are planning to do. If you need to go for tests, have the person who brought you there get some food and drink for themselves. Tell them not to talk about food or bring it back to the cubicle because you may be hungry, but you may not be able to eat.

I once yelled at my poor, dear husband when the doctor had come in. He was only trying to help me by talking to the doctor. I was in pain, cranky, and I told him to leave the cubicle. It was the one and only time that I ever did that to him. Here he was helping, and I was getting mad at him. I am sure he was stressed and nervous too. Sometimes, you just need your own quiet time.

If you must use the restroom or get up for anything, make sure your gown is closed (snapped or tied) in the back. Once while I was getting out of bed, unbeknownst to me, my gown was open.

During one of my emergency room visits, I had severe back pain. A pleasant, thin-framed doctor treated me. He was so kind and very professional in his manner. He looked at my chart and gave me an immediate lidocaine (numbing agent) patch for my back that stops nerves from sending pain signals. It is a local anesthetic that was very cold when applied, but so pain relieving as well. You do not need a prescription, and can purchase them in various drugstores. He noted that I had previous surgery just two weeks prior to going to this ER.

Also, make sure if you are giving a urine sample, that staff should explain fully the instructions, because it is a bit challenging. The sample should be labelled as soon as possible. Try not to leave it in the bathroom. Staff should label the specimen correctly, and immediately proceed to send it off to the lab for testing.

One time I had intense buttock anal pain. No matter what I tried, I had immense pain. I went to a local emergency room in Delaware. It was not busy, and to my surprise was a nice-looking, modern, clean hospital, and they were organized. I was promptly taken in the triage room and told the female nurse why I came to the hospital. She then brought me into an examining room. It also was neat, clean, and tidy. I was greeted by a middle-aged attending physician who wore his glasses on top of his head. He asked me why I was there. I showed him my dilemma and he said,

"Oh yes, these hemorrhoids have to be taken care of promptly."

He medicated me quickly at the local site of discomfort and brought in a very handsome young male nurse. I was in so much agony; however, I remember it was also very embarrassing to have another male individual see my total disaster of a 'cluster of grapes' (as they were called)—a large cluster of hemorrhoids!

Being Admitted

YOU HAVE BEEN GIVEN the glorious news you have to be admitted. Sometimes waiting for a bed could be take a while, or just a short time. There is a lot to do with unit individualized floors when transferring, charting and bed availability. Find out what type of unit you are headed to when being moved from the emergency room. Some are medical floors; some are surgical floors. They are individualized according to what is needed to help you improve. Today, it is not like the days when friends or family could call the hospital to ask about your condition. Because of HIPPA laws for privacy, the friends and family cannot get information. It protects the patient's privacy.

There is frankly nothing better than a private room, but that is not always feasible. I did have both experiences of a private and semi-private room. When I had my children, I was so very incredibly grateful I had private rooms for them. I think all moms should have privacy. It is not a good practice just to pull the curtain and talk about your medical history with another patient in the room, or have visitors in a room while you are trying to rest. It is difficult, on both sides of the bed, to explain things and have someone else overhear the information as well.

I did have the unfortunate experience of sharing a room after I just had major Whipple resection, an extraordinarily complex operation to remove the head of the pancreas, the first part of the small intestine, the gallbladder and the bile duct.

The Whipple procedure may cause many challenges including digestive difficulties for a long time, and it may take a few months to a year to feel relatively normal again. To be honest with you, it did take just about a year. As a nurse, I never actually witnessed one because my specialties were different at the time as an operating room nurse. I was assigned to gynecology, plastic, orthopedic ambulatory surgery. Certain nurses were designated to do those procedures with the surgeons. However, I remember I would cringe as a patient, when it was explained that I needed one. It made my knees weak, my mind and stomach sick to know I had to endure such a complex and long surgery and recovery.

I just could not get any rest because I was in a semi-private room. The older female patient would moan, call the nurse for assistance to get out of bed, and she called her family overseas in the middle of the night. I complained I could not get any rest, and I told my night nurse about the trouble I was having. I needed solitude, sleep, and I truly needed to regroup. I remember thinking I cannot call anyone because it is the middle of the night.

It was quite unsanitary to share a bathroom with another individual. From a nursing point of view, the housecleaning staff usually does a great job taking care of the sanitary conditions of the bathroom. Again, speaking as a nurse, I have noticed there are some patients who do not treat the bathroom as a garbage can, and others who do. As a patient my point of view stays the same, but when you are in pain, I do understand that at times we cannot do much for ourselves, let alone keep the bathroom clean and sanitized for a roommate.

The next day, I spoke to my dear sister Cathy. She is in the healthcare field as well. She was very communicative with the staff and she promised me it would get done with a private room so I could rest. She made some calls to various staff members at the hospital where I was a patient. I was visited by the head nurse and a social worker who helped me immensely. I just told them what I needed and that day I received my private room. The doctor wanted to discharge me, but I said I will go home the next morning. I made the room dark, closed the door and got much needed rest. You must speak up if you are unhappy in any way.

I have also had a forty-two-pound, benign tumor removed, which frankly looked like a watermelon near the ovary. I also had a total abdominal hysterectomy done in the same day. In this procedure, your uterus and cervix will be removed. You may be referred for a hysterectomy because you have uterine, cervical, or ovarian cancer, uterine fibroids, endometriosis, heavy vaginal bleeding, or pelvic pain. Your doctor will explain why you are having the surgery.

Please keep essentials close to your bed. Have your glasses, a pen, paper, hand sanitizer, phone, possibly your phone charger, tissues, your water, and cups nearby. I had beach slippers close to the bed as well for walking around. This way you can reach and not have to ask anyone. If you do need things, ask for things all at once, if possible. It is frustrating not to have something as simple as tissues when you cannot reach it. I used to write things down for patients like a mini grocery list. It is embarrassing when they say, "Oh, I forgot to bring it", and you are waiting. There is a call bell on the side rail of the bed; there is also one in the bathroom as well, if you need it when you ambulate. There are hand sanitizers along the wall, and in the hallways too. Use these sanitizers, as they help keep you from getting a staph infection or other infection that may cause a fever and lengthen your stay.

Nurses do a bedside report in your room. You hear about your day from the nurse's standpoint and all the pertinent information about your progress. I was always adding my two cents as well. I could not help it. I felt it was important to tell them. I have mixed feelings about bedside report. I preferred to speak about the patient at the nurse's desk and then greet the patient.

It is also crucial to take any medications needed for discomfort. The nurses usually have a portable computer and they can tell you when you are due or when you had it last. Oral medications can take a while to work, or sometimes a few minutes. On the other hand, intramuscular and intravenous medications are quicker acting. Try not to refuse or fall behind. This is important if they want you to be walking or using the bathroom or sitting in a chair.

Take notice, to see if there are "white boards" in the room. One is usually on the wall near the foot of your bed. It gives you information about who is going to be your doctor, the names of the day and evening nurses, and includes the date, your diet, and if you are required to have any special test done in addition to any numbers of your medical team, if you need to reach out. It should be updated at each shift.

Talking about each shift, nurses usually work a 12-hour shift and it is a long one. As a nurse for many years, I can personally tell you that it is tiring to say the least. Many days we did not get a chance to eat properly, therefore I would keep healthy snacks in my pockets. While my children were young, I used to fill in short shifts in the schedule. I may have worked a four-or eight-hour shift.

Nutrition—Diet Trays

DEPENDING ON YOUR STATUS, you will be given a diet tray. You may not have ordered what is given but you can ask for something else if it is requested in time, and is possible. If you are on a particular diet (gluten free, low sodium, low calorie), tell them. The food may not be plentiful, and not generally good. One time I was hungry, and I ordered what sounded like a decent tray and when it came, it was so unappealing. I immediately lost my appetite. However, there were times at various hospitals that the food was good.

I asked the female dietary aide who wore both gloves and a cap, but she could not assist, as she was just delivering trays. I then asked my technician who was a noticeably young early twenties, white, and sweet, to see what stash was in their kitchen pantry and refrigerator. They usually have crackers, jelly, peanut butter, cereal, graham crackers, teabags, Jell-O, and coffee packets. I asked her to bring me a few things because I was not eating dinner. I really could have called dietary (nutrition) but I just wanted something small to eat. Occasionally the floor has sandwiches that are made ahead of time too. If you have food brought in from outside of the hospital, you can have it labeled with your name and room number. They can store it in the kitchen refrigerator.

Please be aware you have the right to refuse treatment, or anything for that matter. I was getting continuous blood sticks for blood sugars, but I subsequently refused it after they consistently came back normal. I also refused to have a continuous intravenous still going. It was hurting my arm and they wanted to re-stick me. I was eating, drinking, and using the bathroom. They must have grumbled under their breath, "She is annoying and difficult." Usually the lab technicians come in real early in the morning hours. The doctors and residents come in early as well for bedside check on the patient.

I used to put earplugs in my ears at night to help with the annoying sounds, talking, beeping of machines, etc. It truly did help reduce the external noises during the night. In addition, keep your door closed if possible.

Operating Room

I KNOW, I KNOW; the idea of surgery is frightening. Just to hear those words flying out of your doctor's mouth feels like a death sentence. Surgery, no matter how minor, can be scary as Hell. I know the angst, both professionally and personally.

As a professional nurse, I have been in the room with patients and their attending doctors. While the doctor is explaining the surgery, the look of fear in their eyes tell us just how afraid the patients are. It is our job to help belay those fears by explaining how the surgery will go, and what to expect.

As a patient, however, the nurse in me ran out of the room, and the frightened patient lay in the bed while the attending doctor and the nurse explained the procedure in every detail.

To be honest, I have friends who said to me, "Georgia, you don't do anything small", and my reaction was, "Indeed, and things are usually a bit complicated as well."

They were right. I have had both minor issues with my health, and severe major issues and surgeries. The nurse in me is the one who is writing this book for you; although I am a nurse, I am human, and I know what goes on in the hospital on both sides of the bed. Also, the patient in me has had so many questions. I have such a passion and respect for the operating room, having assisted there too as a nurse. However, when my time came, I was most scared, and the fear led me to think that maybe ignorance is bliss ... but we nurses do appreciate informed patients.

Many times, I had to wait for the scheduled surgery date to arrive, and the waiting game is nerve-wracking and very trying on the body. My brother Patrick, a retired frontline firefighter who was in the World Trade chaos, called or texted me everyday before my surgery and I was moved by his compassion and love.

There are words we all fear—"You need surgery."

Before you are admitted in the facility where you will have the surgery, you will need to get preoperative medical clearance. You may also be required to meet your hospital surgical team. They will give you a detailed information packet to review, depending on the type of surgery.

The hospital staff will tell you what unit you will be going to after surgery. It is usually the recovery room or step-down specialty floor staff that closely monitors your progress and vital signs, but this will be discussed with you ahead of time.

You may also need an electrocardiogram in addition to blood work. The electrocardiogram is a quick, easy and painless procedure that measures your heart's electrical activity. At times they also ask for a chest x-ray just to make sure that your lungs can handle the anesthesia. This essentially means that if the tests come back with all your readings leading to normal or what is normal for you, your doctor will clear you for your surgical procedure. This is vital, especially if you have a pre-existing condition such as heart disease or asthma, or any neurological problems.

There are various types of anesthesia, depending on the type of surgery. For some ambulatory surgeries, the anesthesia is more local, quick-acting and less invasive. For others, the anesthesia is general, in which you are put in a deep sleep. This type of drug can lead to many complications. Ask your doctor or your anesthesiologist questions about this. As a nurse and a patient, I advise you to ask your surgeon: *How long is the procedure, and is it complicated? How long will I stay in the hospital? What kind of incision will I have? Will I have drains put in?*

Before your surgery you will be informed that you cannot wear jewelry, any make-up or have your contact lenses or hearing aid in when you go into the operating room. You can have gel nails or polished nails. On a personal note, ask in the testing unit prior to your surgery date, if you can have your nails done. It may make you feel better to get your hair, nails and toes done. It made me feel good and positive about myself, a must before something so invasive as surgery. During recovery, it may be some time before you can do this.

My sister once said to me when she was admitted for surgery, that she felt she was incarcerated. I thought it was not only funny, but quite true. You may think that is an odd way to think about things when you are in the hospital. Well, either before an ambulatory procedure, or if you are admitted for a while, triage will tell you to remove your clothes, and put them in a white bag. They then ask you to put on a gown, a surgical hat, socks on and sit on the stretcher or bed. Wearing those hospital clothes, one may think they are incarcerated—but it is funny to think about it. Make sure they label your white clothes bag so that it will not get lost. It may come with you to the operating room, or be handed to a family member. You truly are very vulnerable at this point, to say the least.

The pre-operative nurses will take all your vitals (blood pressure and put a white device on you to measure your oxygen saturation. (https://www.healthline.com/health/normal-blood-oxygen-level) A pulse oximeter (pulse ox) is a noninvasive device. A measurement of your blood oxygen is called your oxygen saturation level. Oxygen saturation refers to the amount of oxygen that is in your bloodstream. The body requires a specific amount of oxygen in your blood to function properly. The normal range of oxygen saturation for adults is 94 to 99 percent. Therefore tests are done before, so that your team knows how well you can handle anesthesia.

In addition, you will have to sign a consent form that gives the doctor permission to perform what needs to be done. The hospital will give you multiple documents to fill out before surgery; among these documents are your patient Bill of Rights, and Rights to Privacy. Make sure you fully understand what they will be doing. If you are unsure about something, please ask questions. Once you sign the consent, you are giving the doctor and the hospital your absolute authorization to perform your surgery and comply with your mutual consent agreement.

The day before the procedure, you might have to wash the operative site with an antiseptic soap. It is not common, but I have used it before surgery. You may have an adhesive patch applied on your lower back (sacral area) before surgery called an Allevyn dressing, that helps to prevent fluid buildup before and after surgery. This patch has helped me in the past. It was only given to me once.

So now, you are all ready and tomorrow is the big day. On the day of the surgery you cannot eat; usually by 10:00 pm the night nurse will come in and take your water jug away from you. You ask why? It is because you cannot eat or drink at least 12 hours before surgery. This is to make sure that you do not have a bad reaction to anesthesia, as you may vomit during or after the surgery in recovery, and that could be dangerous.

Once you are identification banded, the team will be asking you repeated questions, and your name and birth date multiple times— It is a system of checks. They want you to be sure you know what is being done. No matter how big or small surgery is, it is surgery no matter 'how you cut it!' Pardon the pun, I just needed to say that.

Believe me, I know what you are thinking right now; It is a scary time at this point. An anesthesiologist will give you an anesthetic once you see your surgeon and the consent is signed. Anesthesia (from Greek without sensation) is a state of controlled temporary loss of sensation or awareness that is induced for medical purposes. It may include some or all of analgesia (relief from or prevention of pain) paralysis (muscle relaxation) amnesia (loss of memory), and unconsciousness. Your body can take up to a week to clear the medications from your system, but most people will notice it much earlier, often after about 24 hours. The risk of dying in the operating room under anesthesia is extremely small for a healthy person with a scheduled procedure. (www.gasdocs.com-FAQ).

PART 2: THE DAY OF YOUR SURGERY

THE MORNING OF YOUR OPERATION comes, and you wake up with much apprehension. As much as your team has prepared you, I know from experience what this pre-anxiety feels like, and uneasy is the only word for it.

Your doctor will meet with you in your room before the procedure, to make sure that you have been prepared with information and an explanation about your surgery; focusing on what you should know before and after. It can be quite scary to say the least. As you lay on your bed and hear these words about anesthesia, IV saline drip, and pain-killers; fear begins to overwhelm you, but this is normal. Just take a deep breath in, and exhale slowly.

Your attending doctor may tell you that the procedure will be three hours or maybe less. But as a nurse, and from my own experience, we must consider all the factors in the process. Surgeries are clocked for time and continuity. Time is scheduled for the anesthesiologist and surgeon to meet with the patient in the holding (pre-op) area before they enter the OR. Then the anesthesiologist will start the IV, and inform the patient that they will feel sleepy as the meds begin to take affect. At the same time, the doctors are diligently scrubbing and sterilizing their hands and arms, while the nurses are prepping the operating room. As the surgeon steps into the room, the circulator nurse will gown the doctor and assist with gloving them. The scrub nurse cleans the operative site and drapes the patient.

There are two functions as a professional nurse in the operating room. One is the scrub nurse, or a technician whose role is scrub person only. The second is a circulating room or circulator nurse.

Registered nurses can do either role, but I preferred circulating and will explain why. Scrub individuals assist the surgeon with handling the instruments and keeping their table in a sterile field and preparing their table for the type of surgery that would be done. They cannot leave their sterile field.

The circulating room nurse is the one that is not 'sterile', but gowns-up the scrub team, assists the anesthesiologist with the patient, and adjusts the lights, music, and temperature control in the room. We did have music, and it was such a calming feeling while we listened. The circulating nurse was the 'runner', so to speak, for instruments, extra trays, or gauzes for drying up the field of fluids, obtaining more sutures, trays, and equipment that may be additionally needed for the scrub team.

The attire worn in an operating room includes scrub top and pants, surgical booties, a surgical mask, and a surgical round stretchable blue hat or a handmade one to stop any hair from dropping in the doctor's or nurse's face during the surgery. I am always intrigued by the handmade scrub caps. And nowadays, I love the handmade surgical masks too.

Once the surgery is completed, the team will begin to remove the surgical drapes, clean up the patient and bring them into recovery where they are given intravenous pain meds and can get much needed post-operative sleep. After a time, the waking up process from anesthesia begins. This is a measure of how the surgery went, if there were any complications. The recovery nurse procures the order to awaken the patient.

I hope I have explained this accurately, because all those factors must be considered before providing a patient with an estimate of the amount of time their operation will take.

I was always intrigued by patients when they were going off to sleep, and either the anesthesiologist or I would ask, "Where would you like to go on a trip?" The patient would begin to answer us as they drifted off to sleep, and would wake up after the surgery continuing what they were saying while going under anesthesia.

Before each of my surgeries, I asked the surgical team not to tell me when I was going to sleep or would feel sleepy. They respected my wishes. I told them just to put the medicine in. I did not like to know I was going to sleep. If ordered by your surgeon, you may receive intravenous preoperative antibiotics for prophylactic purposes.

When I was a circulating nurse, it would be frustrating at times if the instrument or trays did not come up quick enough from the central supply room and the doctors would be repeatedly asking for it. Generally, you counted on your team to be efficient with the type of surgery and not show insecurity as a scrub team member. Some doctors could easily pick that up. I had to remind them a few times to be patient or be nice, especially when working with them on a frequent basis.

I genuinely enjoyed being a circulating nurse because I took pride in taking care of the patient first and foremost. The operating room is a very technical area, and I love the technical aspect of the machines. You had to have eyes all over to make sure everyone was safe and happy.

I always had a favorite line: "No rush", or "No problem", that I would say to reduce the stress factor in the operating room, and for my team members. I would also joke around to lighten the mood too.

A few times—well, more than a few times—if I were annoyed with the surgeon, I would pull hard and tie their gowns real tight. As a circulator I was permitted to leave the room, and if I was angry, I would step out and curse under my breath to relieve tension, especially if the surgeon was not acting professionally or pleasantly to the team.

Quite often I worked alongside my good friend, whom I also commuted with, and she loved to scrub. One day she was not sure what was in her syringe on her sterile field, and she asked me if I knew what it was. I told her to just shoot the clear fluid on the wall to get rid of it, and reload with what was requested. You can have saline solution or lidocaine numbing medicine on the sterile field. I started to chuckle, and I had to contain myself because my eyes were tearing with laughter. To this day, I remember thoroughly enjoying working with her. She was a funny, smart, friend who had shiny brunette hair and we exchanged much laughter. We were often called the 'A-Team' by fellow surgeons. I saw the look in their eyes when they saw us together prepping the room. We worked together about eleven years, until she moved on and worked exclusively for a plastic surgeon.

Post Operative Room— Recovery Room

FOR THE MOST PART, you will wake up sleepy, but it is expected. You may not remember too much after the anesthesia. You will then be transferred to a recovery room to get your vitals taken repeatedly and a nurse will give you warmth, pain relief and good care. They have come up with great ideas to ward off any nausea ahead of time and it is given in the operating room. Who wants to throw up afterwards? They will observe for any drains, look at your operative site and bandage and read any orders specific to your needs. When the effect of the medicine wears off, the numbed part of the body will return to normal. Depending on which type of anesthesia was used, complete recovery may take four to eight hours (Allina Health patient education).

I once had a very pleasant surprise after I was wheeled into the recovery room. I looked up and my attending surgeon was holding my hand. She was in her mid-thirties, about five feet seven inches tall, and she would frequently adjust her silver metal eyeglasses. She had just performed a procedure to remove my annoying hemorrhoids. They were gross and I needed it done.

She said, "Georgia, everything went well." She held my hand for quite some time. I felt it was very reassuring. She probably felt bad because I did cry very much before I went into the operating room due to knowing too much. Whatever the reason it was, it was a kind and memorable gesture, and will have always be a lasting memory of kindness by a physician.

You may offered a Patient Controlled Medication (PCA) pump, which is a handheld unit. This is a benefit because the patient can self-administer their pain medication such as morphine or codeine, by the way of a click of a button. You cannot overdose because the parameters are ordered and preset. This is given for a short time, because they want to advance you to oral medications. Too much of the PCA medication can cause the bowels to slow up as well. If you hear the machine beeping, the narcotic medication may need to be replenished, or it could be the battery may be low if it is not plugged in and it needs to be changed by the nurse.

You may be discharged after the recovery period. It may be considered same day surgery, or you may just stay overnight. Perhaps you may stay a few days or a week or so. It depends on the doctor, surgery and how you progress.

I will never ever forget one experience I had while in the step-down unit. It was late at night, and after being transferred and hooked up, my vitals started to change out of the normal levels. I usually cannot see far, but I was surprised I could see the numbers so clearly. The beeping of the machines went off on a constant basis. The numbers were out of normal range for me. A kind, calm, and very professional nurse with dark short hair came by and looked at the vitals. She was a superb nurse; she saw how quite concerned I was about the numbers on the screen and the repeated beeping signals. She said those famous words, "Trust me."

I said, "What does it all mean?"

She said in a calm voice, "It is indicating sepsis protocol."

Sepsis is the body's extreme response to an infection. It is a life-threatening medical emergency. Sepsis happens when an infection you already have—in your skin, lungs, urinary tract, or somewhere else—triggers a chain reaction throughout your body. It is quite serious and must be treated immediately with antibiotics. (www.cdc.gov › sepsis). There was an alert on the computer screen. That was all I needed to hear was sepsis.

She said," I am going to call the doctor and we are going to assess the situation." Very professionally and calmly she again repeated, "Trust me."

She called the resident and the doctor said, "Georgia, you have had a good urine output and no fever, but we will do the blood draw in the morning."

I tried to close my eyes and sleep, but I kept peeking at the screen. The early morning hours arrived and they drew my blood. I had no recollection of that, but I did hear her say all the tests are normal. I was over the moon with joy. Again, it is the little things that matter most in life. She was truly an angel and I felt secure and blessed she was my night nurse. I will never forget her or the incidence that occurred.

It is usually loud in the recovery room. You will hear multiple sounds including machines beeping and people talking. The lights will seem bright. Once you wake up enough, they will get your family in for a brief visit. You will have tubes in, for example a urine catheter tube to prevent you from having to go to the bathroom right after surgery. There will have oxygen and an intravenous and anything else discussed ahead of time. The nurse will take your vital signs and medicate you for pain relief. I have had many recovery nurses; although I do not remember their names, but I truly respect them and the unit they work on.

If you have had abdominal surgery, an abdominal binder may be fastened around your tummy. The binder helps secure and hold the stomach with added reinforcement. It is a long thick white band that has Velcro to help adjust the size according to the patient and when you are in bed or ambulating. You can take this home to for continued supportive use. Be aware that when you cough and/or laugh, it will hurt; please hold your stomach with a pillow, as this will cut down on the pain. This is crucial to avoid splitting the incision.

Take note that there will be sequential boots on your feet and legs to help with circulation while you are in bed. These are a great device to prevent any circulation problems. The nurse puts them on both of your legs and activates the machine to help with circulation. Once you are ambulating more, they will remove them.

I love portable handheld computers. The nurse will scan your bracelet and then the medication to be given. It stores your information and lets the nurse know what must be given and when the next dose is to be dispersed. It also prevents mistakes, because if it is the wrong medication, or patient, it will either make a weird buzz sound, or prevent you from proceeding forward.

You may have drains in as discussed before surgery. One is a small Penrose drain that helps remove fluid from the operative area. There is also what is called a Jackson Pratt plastic drain or drains as well. They have long tubes that go inside the body and look like grenades on the outside. These must be drained by the nurse and logged, as to how much liquid is draining along with color. For most patients and for me, it is a challenge to walk around with the binder and drains. Many times it was very frustrating and hard to sleep on my back.

When I had my second abdominal hernia surgery, the doctor explained to me that a mesh (a material made of Hydopolyproplene synthetic plastic which can be absorbed or non-absorbed) would be inserted to help secure the abdominal wall that remains there permanently. This device is a foreign body, but it is highly effective to help maintain and to secure together the abdominal wall. It should not hurt, and you do not see it.

The site looked quite deformed, and I was mortified to look at it before it was done. I had multiple bumps throughout my stomach; since I used to ski, I pictured them looking just like ski moguls.

Once you meet the recovery room criteria, you will be transferred to a unit to recover. It sometimes takes a while to get there due to charting, bed availability and someone to transfer you etc. This will be the unit you will most likely be on until you are discharged. Once they move you, please support your incision with a pillow if you can. The stretcher does go over speed bumps in the hallway, and the bed shakes a bit as you are moved.

Keep your hands inside the side rails too for added safety. Most of the time the intern moving you will make sure that you do. Wheelchairs are a great source of transportation to get around the hospital as well but try to hold your incision, because the ride could get bumpy as well.

Surgical Unit—Continuance of Recovery

THIS IS THE SURGICAL FLOOR or unit you will probably be on until you go home. You may or may not be in a private room and not remember too much. Just rest and relax at this time. Visitors are great, and it is nice to see familiar faces, but it can also make you tired. I am indeed blessed to have had my family at my bedside taking turns visiting. I tried very hard to stay awake. They traveled out of state to see me. I am forever and truly grateful they were there. I am sure they were both worried and relieved to see I did well, and the surgery was over too. They were supportive to me and provided massive support, gifts, phone calls, texts, and prayers while I recovered.

The first day post-operative is quite crucial. Most of the tubes you have in, especially the urine catheter, will be removed. It does not hurt when it comes out. Your post-op nurse will measure your urine output by placing a 'hat' (a urine receptacle) in the toilet to collect the sample and check on both the color and the amount.

I cannot stress enough the importance of being medicated for pain before you get up. Take the medication even if your pain level is low. Remember, the head of the bed can be raised; I recommend utilizing this. You should also move towards the edge of the bed and push off with the raised side rail. A nurse may help you up, but this is also another way especially if you are alone in the room and need to get up. You can also raise the bed up and down depending on the height you want by pushing a button on the side rail.

I have had a specialist surgical attending doctor yell at me in front of his staff, when I was a patient. My immediate family was present when he was giving me orders and I was mortified.

"Georgia you are not getting up enough or walking after this most major abdominal surgery. You know how vital it is to do so."

I said, "How am I supposed to know? I didn't see the orders."

As a nurse and a patient, it is crucial to ambulate when you are allowed and are hospitalized. It is helpful in many ways, especially in getting your system back on track, and encouraging the digestive system to work again.

Gas pains are very painful, and can sometimes travel to the shoulders. One time the pain caused by gas pockets in my stomach were so bad. I remember saying to my sister Cathy, who walked with me in the hallway,

"I am not going back to that operating room!"

I could not get my system to work. I kept trying and nothing was happening. Finally, I just watched a movie with my family and low and behold, my system woke up and the pain disappeared. If you are having trouble passing flatus (gas), they can give you something to help it along. Walking really helps, and peppermint tea or a gas relief tablet may be ordered too. They may have tea on the unit. A heating pad may help alleviate the pain as well.

If you cannot shower, you can just wash up. They have multi-function bath wipes. I have the pleasure of once getting them heated in the microwave and using them on my body. They also have regular ones as well. Dry shampoo, sold in drugstores, is a great product for freshening up your hair. Brushing your teeth and washing up is a great feeling. You should try to get request a new gown for yourself, if you have not already done so, as it might have been soiled or wet, or simply dirty from surgery and recovery room. It is not a bad idea to bring your own pillow or blanket as an added comfort, if you wish.

Just be careful with your phone, glasses, or anything else you may leave in the bed. You don't want anything to get lost in the linens when they are changed. Also, don't leave any of your personal items on the diet trays, as they may also be taken away with the tray.

I cannot stress enough how vital it is to use the incentive spirometer at your bedside. Make sure you know how to use this device. It helps you expand your lungs while you are in bed, and helps you if you are not actually doing it due to your surgery. I had a young, fast-walking resident who was very good and effective at her job. She said, "I want you to do this now!"

She gave me the number she wanted me to reach for the incentive spirometer to work effectively. It is for your benefit. It can prevent possibly any lung infection from occurring while you are immobile. If you cannot do the amount asked at once, then do it in smaller more frequent increments like I did.

If your room is too cold or hot, it can either be adjusted in your room, or by engineering. I have had to ask to have someone come in to adjust the temperature to my liking. Try to keep the door closed if possible, to keep both the noise down, and the proper temperature so you will be comfortable.

There may be a dressing over your incision. It may be white with lots of tape or a clear plastic one. Either way there will be pulling of hair and skin when it is removed. Try to take a deep breath at this point. You may notice, as I did, this purple glue on your incision. I never had it before, but it looked a bit odd. It is a waterproof glue sealant on top of the incision. I was glad I had it. It will eventually peel with your help, just like you would peel super glue off your fingers. I felt it was an additional sealant.

Once you start to progress and your tummy starts to wake up and make sounds, you will be advanced in your diet. You can ask the nurse if you can have outside food and drinks brought in by family.

Another good practice is to pull around the curtain near your bedside. You can draw it all the way around your bed for added privacy. I did this sometimes just to shut the world out. It also helped to prevent people from entering the room and seeing things that you might not want them to observe. The drapes vary in style and neutral colors, but they all have the same purpose. They just pull around your bed area to enhance your need for privacy.

Just be prepared that the first day after surgery may a bit of a challenge. You usually have experienced pain due to mobility and have a need for pain medications. They may have you sit in a chair for a while too. It usually gets better with each day. Take it slow and easy. Walk and take your medications to help alleviate any discomfort. I tried so hard with my last surgery to do all this. I was able to leave the hospital sooner than what my doctor had told me. I was proud of myself for working hard at this.

If possible, have comfortable clothes and shoes to wear when you are discharged and can return home. You may still have a bandage on or have some swelling. You will need someone to take you home.

Discharge

THIS IS TRULY A GREAT TIME, when you can go home to your own place. Once you are seen by your doctor to make sure all the requirements have been met, then you are good to go home. If you feel you are not ready, stay additional days if it is possible. Discuss your concerns to the staff.

You will receive post-operative discharge instructions that the staff will read to you. Make sure that if you do not understand something, ask them. It is particularly important to understand each segment of your instructions. They would provide you with things to look for if the incision site got infected or you did not feel well afterwards. You will also get a date when you will see your doctor in the office. They may also ask you to call the doctor's office. Check if it's normal for your dressing to soil and when it should be taken off unless they remove it in the hospital. Even if I knew what to expect on the instructions, I listened attentively, and asked questions to reconfirm what was being explained.

If you need gloves for anything, they can be given to you along with tape and or extra white gauze dressings if it needed to be changed. Make sure you are told how often to change and remove them. You may or may not get a prescription ordered. I set up in my phone, text messages to alert me if medication is ready for pick up or delayed from the pharmacy.

It is advisable to wash the clothes and wipe down all the items you brought to the hospital with wipes. Don't forget to wipe your phone and eyeglasses, and anything else you brought in or used as well. Proper hand washing is always important, especially during, and after COVID-19.

Before you leave the hospital, they will ask you if you need a visiting nurse or help at home. It is to make sure you can get all the help you may need. Sometimes social workers provide you with the resources needed to help you with this process.

Please rest when you get home as much as possible. It will take a long time to get your stamina and strength back. You may get tired just from making breakfast, or taking a shower. I felt that was always the case with me. It may take weeks or even months to feel yourself again. Try to do activities in increments or postpone doing them until you feel better.

One time, I did have these Jackson Pratt grenade-shaped plastic drains in my surgical site and had to lie on my back for over two weeks before they were removed. It was not at all easy to say the least. I could not turn to either side because I was afraid that I would occlude the bulbs that were draining. I had unbelievably bad, sleepless nights and therefore I took periodic naps during the day. I had a binder on as well to hold them up. It was a terrific feeling to be rid of them once they were removed. I felt I was free!

As for weight loss, you may see it right away or as time goes by. I weighed more in the hospital due to the accumulation of fluids etc. You may have to adjust your eating habits to smaller, more frequent meals and not be overeating. Drinking water is crucial as well, as previously discussed. You may or not have swelling in your hands and feet. This will go away when you walk, drink fluids, and when you use the restroom. After a bit of time, I did lose a good amount of weight (about seventy-five pounds) due to the type of surgery I had done. It might also be from not eating too much before and after surgery as well. An older woman who lives in my community once said to me, "Wow, you lost a lot of weight!" She then proceeded to say, "But I do not like the way you did it."

I simply had no choice in the matter, and I had nothing to say.

If you have pets, please be aware to avoid having them jump on you and near your incision. Pets mean well, but just be careful. They are curious and concerned for us and might not be aware of what is going on. They are so precious, and they love us unconditionally. I love them too and it touches me to have them care for us in their own unique way. My Maine Coon cat Nala (a male with a female name), would jump on me and tentatively go to my incision site.

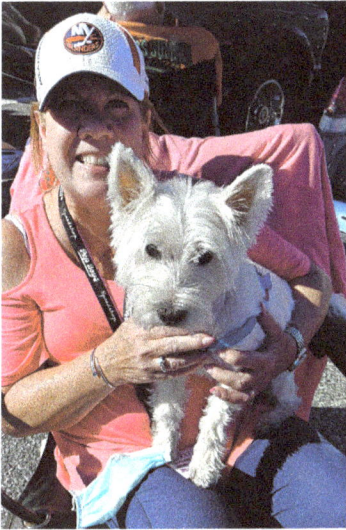

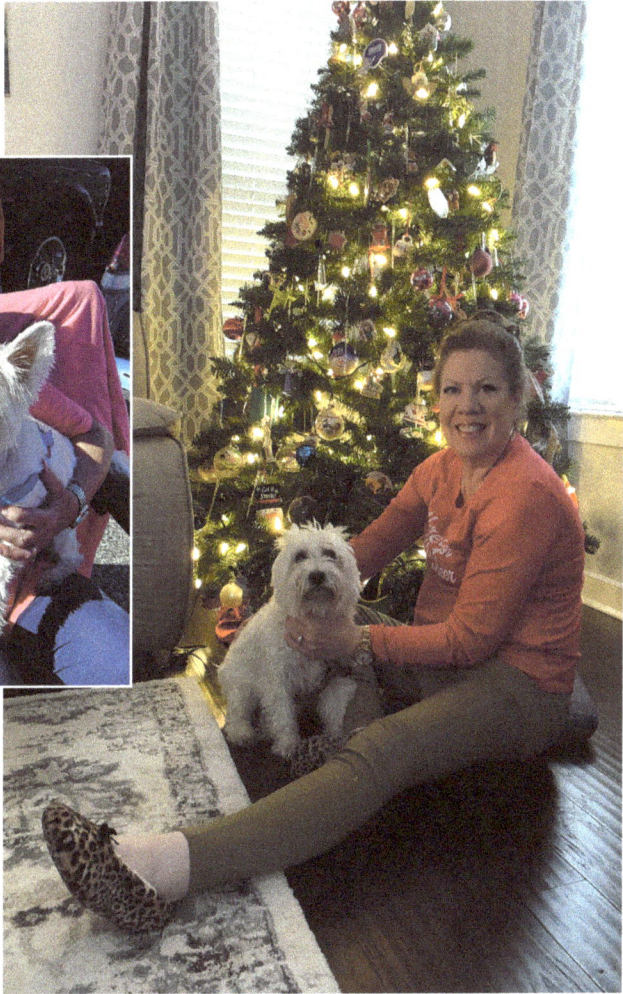

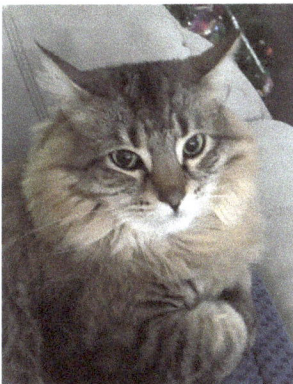

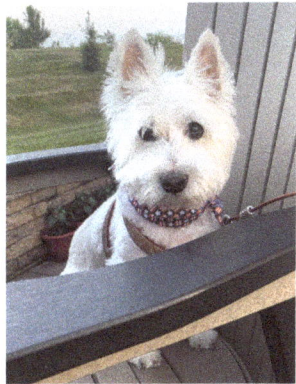

Above left:
True Paw Friend

Above:
True Paw Friend

Left: My curious and
loyal cat Nala.

Right:
My loyal Buddy
(13 years old when
photo was taken).

My dog Buddy, a Westhighland terrier, would follow me everywhere as well.

Keep an eye on your temperature if you feel warm. If you experience chills, excess pain, or have a temperature, please call the doctor immediately. Keep your post-operative instructions and doctor's number nearby to access them. Although a fever technically is any body temperature above the normal of 98.6°F (37°C), in practice a person is usually not considered to have a significant fever until the temperature is above 100.4°F (38°C). The temperature is measured with a thermometer. It is shaken down after use and wiped with alcohol for disinfecting. It is significant to know if you have a fever because it may be indicative of an infection.

It might or might not happen, but I experienced quite a lot of hair loss. It was so disheartening and scary. I could not believe it frankly, what I was witnessing in my hairbrush and in the shower. I tried many hair volume treatments. I started to take biotin vitamins and used organic volume shampoos. It took some time, which seemed like an eternity, before it stopped happening. I could not believe it when I say, I saw my scalp—and I have had very thick hair. It took a few months for me to see a difference in the thickness.

Gratitude for the Doctors and Staff

I AM FOREVER AND SINCERELY thankful to all the staff members who have assisted me immensely throughout the years. I am also grateful for all you have done for me in any sort of way to help me. You made a difference and I so appreciate it.

When I was in New York, I had a nurse practitioner who was in her late twenties at the time, an attractive woman who would wear dark rimmed glasses that matched her shiny brunette hair. She always dressed very professional and very chic. She helped me with my ears when I had major wax build up. She kept trying hard; she spent a lot of time with me and I could see her determination with trying to help me. I was so thankful that I was able to hear and did not have to go to an ear specialist to get treated. She was thorough at her job and many times I would see her for appointments. My doctor was not available, but I knew in my heart, she was more than capable. I even went to her when I had a problem with my right kidney. She collaborated with my primary doctor about what she found regarding the pain I was exhibiting at the time.

Once I had excruciating back pain while I was on a softball field and got quite dizzy. It was a humid, hot day, and it was the championship game for my daughter's team. The event was stressful, and loud and this was an important game for the girls. I got up from a sitting position and my head spun, and I experienced a wave of light-headedness.

I remembered it very clearly. I did not want to make a scene, but I summoned an anesthesiologist, and friend I knew after the game. I told him my symptoms and he then stated to me, "I am calling an ambulance."

I said, "Please, just give me a few minutes."

I finally came around and with the help of my husband and my friend, I was ushered to the car. The air conditioner was blasting, and I said I would be okay. I made an appointment the next morning. Yes, I am quite tough and stubborn. I felt a bit better that evening except for some pain in my right lower back. I made an appointment with my trusty nurse practitioner, as my primary doctor was unavailable. She ran tests and then forwarded the result to my primary physician.

My doctor sent me for a sonogram. I had it done locally, and when the technician hobbled in with her crutches, I got quite a deliverance of bad news. She was very talkative and explained how she hurt her foot. We talked and talked and then there was dead silence. I knew right away something was not right. She scrambled out the room and said she would be right back. The next minute an older technician or radiologist came in and stared at the screen. They were both speechless. I kept saying, "Is everything alright?" The technician then proceeded to explain this massive tumor on the screen that took up the entire computer monitor. I jumped up and then felt a wave of nausea take over. They both looked like they were in shock. I called my husband, Don. He came right away because I could not drive home. My head was spinning around in circles. I thought I was doomed.

Subsequently, I was hit with big, shocking, and unexpected news. My primary doctor called me, and stated I had a huge football-like tumor on my right kidney.

Angiomyolipoma (AML) is a benign renal neoplasm composed of fat, vascular, and smooth muscle. I was told that it was massive but thank God it was benign. However, I did lose my right kidney in the process. The tumor was massive, and the poor kidney was hidden. The doctor said they both had to come out together. Initially I was saddened to think I would lose a perfectly normal right kidney, but you can live a normal life with one kidney. They diagnosed it quickly due to large size it was. I knew ahead of time what I had.

I was extremely dizzy due to the bleeding of the vessels that were starting to leak and spurt out blood. I was immediately admitted because my EKG was slightly abnormal due to low potassium levels. The levels had to be corrected before they proceeded forward. I was given intravenous potassium that burned like a hot coil in my arm. One staff nurse diluted it, or slowed the drip down.

I had a low blood count (anemic low red blood cells). Although it was quite low, I did not require a blood transfusion. I went home with that number and the doctor said eat well and it will improve. I was so tired, but it did get better over time. It took a couple of weeks to begin building up my strength and stamina. My mom came and stayed with me to help me with the kids, laundry, phone calls, and cooking while my husband worked. Rest and proper nutrition, and foods high in iron helped me to recover from this low blood deficiency.

Thank God, I had my fabulous primary doctor back in New York. He was a six-foot tall, clean shaven physician, who looked like a teddy bear and wore metal rimmed glasses. He had the friendliest eyes you can imagine. During the years that I knew him, his weight would fluctuate but as it neared the end of my visits, he was pleasantly trim, and he was proud of it.

He was always jovial and upbeat when I had to see him. He cheered me up many times and just made me smile. He always had a huge warm smile that was consistent throughout the years. I was never embarrassed to ask him anything. He reminded me of my dear dad with his easy-going demeanor. My dad was the same height and had this friendly happy-go-lucky personality. He helped guide me to an exceptionally good general surgeon. I usually went in for appointments and I would say to him what I thought may be wrong with me, like bronchitis, etc.

He once said, "You make my job easy." He took great pride in his work.

I trusted him when he told me things.

I once asked him, "Would you send your family member to the doctor you are referring me to?"

When I had the big issue with my right kidney and when all the tests were back, he referred me to the right person. He loved his job. He really is the sweetest and kindest physician I have ever met. One of his major accomplishments is that he is considered a highly-rated internal medicine specialist in New City, Rockland County, NY. He is affiliated with one hospital in upstate NY and has been in practice for more than 20 years and is still practicing today. He shares an office with other doctors and nurse practitioners and performs physicals. One in every four doctors in the United States are internists.

I am grateful that the doctor referred me to a urology specialist, when I had the massive kidney tumor. This attending general surgeon would ultimately do my surgery for my football sized tumor and removal of my right kidney. I immediately met him while I was being hospitalized to correct the low potassium level. He was in his mid-fifties, and had a full head of white hair and dashing blue eyes. He was both soft-spoken and very calm in his demeanor. He remarked about my New York Mets bag I had on the chair. He said, with a huge smile, he was a fan too.

Right before surgery, he told me that the tumor was huge but benign and my kidney needed to be removed. They could see it was not due to the structure and enormity of the tumor that it could be differentiated. I was happy it was not cancerous.

This was a huge surgical procedure and it was one of the biggest I initially had undergone. When I was in the surgical intensive care unit, my family, my adorable son Ryan, and beautiful daughter Jillian came to visit me. I do not remember too much but what I do remember was my family taking turns coming in to see me.

When my children to came in to see their mommy, Jillian said, "Mom I do not want to leave you." She insisted she wanted to continue to stay.

I then heard my caring husband Don say, "We need to go."

I put my tired arm out and said to him, "Don, let her stay."

Jillian did not want to leave, and she sat down with me in my groggy state. It was sad to see a nine-year-old have to witness

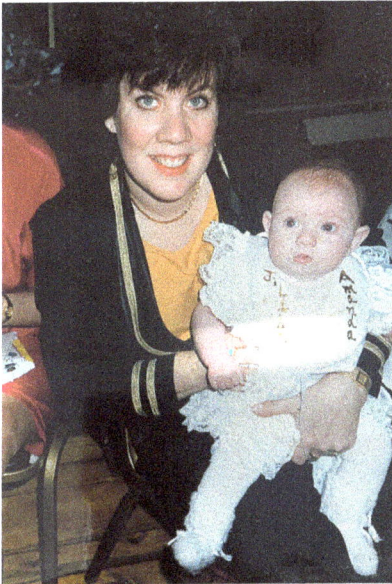
My darling Jill.

seeing me in a hospital bed with tubes and monitors attached to me. It boggles me to wonder what went through their minds when they saw me. I have tears as I am writing this. For children, it must have been so frightening for them.

After my family left, a small-framed nurse came on duty. In my sleepy state, she was trying to turn me and remarked with a sigh and a grumble about my size. I tried to help her, but I felt sad that she was so rude in her remarks. I thought about the positives and how I made it through hours of surgery, and they stated the 'football' was a benign cyst-like tumor. What I was initially unhappy about was the fact that my normal right kidney had to be removed. The doctor said it needed to be removed because the tumor was bleeding and he could not visualize the kidney and felt this was the safest route.

After a few days in the surgical unit, I was transferred to a small private room on a surgical floor. The hospital was immaculate, with fresh paint, upgraded floors, and renovated rooms throughout. I was introduced to a male nurse who seemed busy at the time, but was both professional and friendly. He helped me with ambulating and medicating me when I needed it and was prompt at his response time when I called. What followed next was another episode of not being able to pass gas. It was so disheartening and most frustrating. I walked the halls and took the required medicine, but my system decided to take a nap. The pain then escalated, and it seemed like hours later that I returned to a normal state.

For my initial hernia surgery, I was referred to a general surgeon for a huge abdominal hernia that I noted to my primary physician. He was a thin, tall doctor in his mid-fifties, who had brown hair and wore small dark glasses. He had a matter of fact disposition, and was a bit distant in his approach—no warm or fuzzy feeling. However, I knew he was highly intelligent and had good credentials. He was a general surgeon with over thirty-three years experience. A surgical specialist is a doctor who has additional training in certain areas of expertise. He had special training in laparoscopic, hernia, breast diseases and gastrointestinal surgery. He saw my stomach and right away told me what needed to be done.

He also looked at my stomach and said, "You have a big stomach."

Talk about being mortified. His office manager made up for his rudeness and curt behavior by going out of her way to being extra friendly and very caring She was receptive to my needs and was non judgemental. I actually asked her is he normally rude? I did think to myself, should I just go to someone else? Doctors may not all be nice, but bedside manners are important too. I overlooked it and moved forward with my decision to get it fixed.

I had a second abdominal hernia repair one way before my Whipple procedure and one after. I was told I needed a second one in order to maintain and the adequateness and stability of my abdominal wall. The second procedure was done in Delaware.

My hernia specialist, who had just mentioned he turned forty, was a handsome doctor with an athletic build, and a thin and trimmed facial mustache and beard. He is was both outgoing and had a friendly disposition, and always greeted me with a handshake (before this coronavirus outbreak).

One of the most endearing things he said to me was, "You are my star patient."

He also continued to say, "You are like the bionic woman."

I chuckled at that and thought, "Wow, is that what he thinks of me? I am almost 60!"

It gave me such a boost and made me quite proud. I walked around that day with my head held high. He truly is a great doctor who is always calm, cool, and friendly. He answered all my questions, and there were many of them. I will always be grateful to him. I was also pleased with the neatness of the incision. He helped clean up the previous scar. The good doctor is Section Chief of General Surgery and medical director of the hernia center, with special interests in complex abdominal wall hernia repair and wall reconstruction as well as all aspects of hernia related care. He is certified by the American Board of Surgery. I was extremely impressed by his humbleness and his achievements. He is both proficient in Laparoscopic and open hernia surgery, and has over four plus years training as a general surgeon and with additional training in Robotic Surgery. He was very thorough in his description of what needed to be addressed.

At times, I felt that the information I received from him was too much. He meant well though. The hospital was two hours from my house, but we did not mind because it was so well worth it.

Hernia mesh is made of synthetic materials which come in woven or non-woven forms or a combination of both. The most popular types of surgical mesh are made from polypropylene, a synthetic plastic non-absorbable mesh that will remain in the body indefinitely as a permanent implant reinforced to the repaired hernia.

Terry Turner has been writing articles and producing news broadcasts for more than 25 years. He covers FDA policy, proton pump inhibitors, and medical devices such as hernia mesh, IVC filters, and hip and knee implants. An Emmy-winning journalist, he has reported on health and medical policy issues before Congress, the FDA, and other federal agencies. Some of his qualifications include:

- American Medical Writers Association (AMWA) and The Alliance of Professional Health Advocates member

- Centers for Disease Control and Prevention Health Literacy certificates

- Original works published or cited in Washington Examiner, Med Page Today and The New York Times

- Appeared as an expert panelist on hernia mesh lawsuits on the BBC

The article states: "A hernia is a protrusion of intestinal abdominal fat *(Dr. Scott Laker weight loss and hernia repair) (momentum) commonly through a weakness in the muscle wall."

"The incidence of a person developing some type of hernia in their lifetime is approximately 10 percent. One million hernia repairs are performed annually in the United States. Approximately 750,000 are inguinal hernia. Although the tenants of hernia repair appear to be well established, surgical technique continues to be refined in hopes of providing a repair with complete durability, minimal pain and elimination of infection and other potential complications" (Dr. Scott Laker Hernia and weight loss surgery).

The obstetrical gynecology attending physician was both a colleague at a Westchester hospital where I had worked for eleven years, and who eventually became my doctor. Standing hardly five feet tall, she is a petite powerhouse of a doctor; a short-haired woman with big hazel eyes that could say a thousand words without ever speaking. I rarely saw her wear pants. She wore cute stylish dresses and dress scrub attire too. I respected her amazing mind and her physical strength as well as her expertise with her baby deliveries despite how tiny she was in stature. She is in her late fifties and has worked many years at this hospital, in the field of obstetrics and gynecology.

I had been going to a male physician for many years for gynecology. He was a sweet man, but not aggressive with treating my heavy monthly cycles. He repeatedly asked me if I was taking vitamins. He safely delivered my daughter. He was very competent and patient with Jillian's delivery. He was not phased in the least bit. He has since retired from his field of expertise. I had suffered for many years, and I just wanted him to treat my crazy menstrual cycles.

When it got out of control, I asked my powerhouse doctor and colleague to help me with a resolution. She sent me for a sonogram, also called an ultrasound; an imaging test that uses sound waves to create pictures of organs, tissues, or other structures within the body. It was a quick, painless procedure. After the results were back, she informed me what needed to be addressed.

She grabbed me one night while we were working and told me I needed a uterine ablation procedure to help me with my issue. She explained what the image on the sonogram disclosed, and it was a decent size fibroid, and my uterine lining was thick.

She explained the procedure in detail what needed to be done and I scheduled it quickly to get this in gear. I did the necessary requirements before surgery and faxed over my previous records to her office. I had it scheduled at the hospital I worked in and was admitted under my maiden name to be a private matter.

The uterine ablation was a heated balloon placed in the uterus and it would expand. It would destroy and ablate the lining of the uterus which is called the endometrium. The goal of this is to reduce the menstrual flow.

When it was time for surgery, the nurses were outgoing and friendly. It was not done on my unit, but on the ambulatory surgical unit. I was scheduled for same day surgery. All went well and I was thrilled I could listen to my music going into the operating room. I had asked my doctor and she said it was fine. I was delighted to know I could be satisfied after it was completed. For months and years that followed, it served me greatly, both physically and personally. I wish I had done this sooner because it would have made life much easier.

There were frankly no issues afterwards and we continually respected each other. I was so pleased she took care of my annoyance. I even talked with one of my closest and dearest friends to get it done due to her same repeated issues. I worked for her for many years until I transferred to another hospital for employment. I just saw her for my annual checkups. I would go back to my former hospital those times because that is where she practices. She is currently still working, and I am sure doing what she does best especially delivering babies!

A New Life

MANY YEARS LATER as we were closing in on retirement and looking for a place to live, I had noted my stomach becoming larger. I thought it was either part of the aging process, another large hernia, or menopause kicking-in at full speed. I was too busy with retiring and deciding where to move, selling our house, and trying to relocate. My health took a back seat, and we finally moved to Delaware. We had no idea who to go to for doctors. We spoke to several neighbors and were told it was a long waiting process to see a doctor here, partly due to the major influx of people who moved there in their retirement life.

It wasn't until I experienced some intense stomach pain that I knew something was amiss. I initially thought that the abdominal hernia was again causing me havoc. The pain intensified and I was scared, but I knew I needed to go to the emergency room. My family urged me to go to get examined. I went to a local hospital that had a busy emergency room department.

Once the results were back, the doctor that I had been assigned went off duty. A new doctor came in and she stood at the foot of my bed telling me my results. She looked very stern and I did not like the fact that she was at the end of my stretcher. She was a short, stocky physician in her mid-thirties, with long unkempt blondish hair.

I simply asked her, "Doctor, please come up to the side of my stretcher and tell me what you need to say." She proceeded, and stood there with her arms crossed, which was quite intimidating for someone who was terrified of the results.

She continued, "Mrs. Murawski, you have a tumor that has encompassed your entire stomach."

Everything and every fear I had came back like a flood of water I thought would drown me.

I did not like her approach, but subsequently she guided me to the right physicians who would ultimately save me at a different hospital. I had to drive two hours from my house to see specialists, but it was worth every minute. She referred me to the right doctors/surgeons.

I immediately was given an appointment with a gynecology and oncology specialist who was again two hours away in a large well-established hospital. He was a short, humble doctor in his early forties, and had both a caring and cheerful demeanor. I became even more anxious was when I was in the room being questioned by his female residents, as they would periodically look at each other. I tried to figure out what they both were doing when they heard my history.

I eventually said, "You are both making me more nervous," took a deep nervous breath, and I blurted out, "I feel like I am doomed."

He immediately replied, "Oh no!"

That was his way and he did it without realizing it. I was then led to his large open windowed office that had multiple certifications, plaques and most of all, his beautiful family pictures displayed.

He told us, "You need one more CT scan to see if there was anything else that may be an issue."

He said, "Mrs. Murawski, you have a huge tumor near your ovary that will be removed along with having a total abdominal hysterectomy, which will also be removed with your gallbladder and appendix as a preventative measure."

I had the appointment made very quickly and I took care of the test promptly. The next morning, I received a call from the doctor — this time he almost knocked me to the floor. I felt like I was hit with a ton of bricks. I could not focus at this point.

He told me, "We think that in the scan we saw something near your pancreas."

I shockingly replied, "Doc, did you say pancreas?"

He said, "Yes."

I stopped him from going on and I asked Don to get the phone and the rest of the information from the call. I truly needed rescuing at this point. I said some prayers and asked God to spare me. I just wanted a simple life, that was all. I did not want to leave this world yet.

Again, I have tears when reminiscing about this most scary time in my life. I cried my eyes out that day and could not regroup. To me, it was a total disaster, and I could see it no other way.

That day was absolutely one of the scariest moments of my life due to the initial diagnosis. I had called my mom and she was trying her best to be encouraging.

Mom said, "There are many updated technologies, Georgia. Don't lose hope."

I remembered one of my other sisters called me, and I just cried more and said to her, "Each time, I go over a higher hurdle and it is getting harder and harder to jump over them." I felt my breath catch in my chest. "How much could one person endure and still be standing?"

I was constantly getting knocked down, and repeatedly got hit in the face with bricks. I honestly thought I had limited time on this earth, and it made me very sad, and quite miserable. I could not think of anything else. I had lost my dear dad to melanoma, (the deadliest form of skin cancer) years back at the age of fifty-four and I thought, oh wow, I am going to die young too.

The doctor also said I needed to see a gastroenterologist to be able to pinpoint the exact diagnosis of the tumor. This doctor was to meet with me in the office, but I suggested instead of going to his office, to just do the endoscopy to determine what I had specifically. I was booked as an add-on the following week.

I entered the endoscopy suite and waited very patiently to meet the doctor; he was thin and extremely tall, about six foot five to be exact, and is in his late thirties. Both my husband and my daughter were there too. I was so sad because all I wanted was for my family of four to remain a family of four, not three. Although it was late in the day and I had not eaten, I was ready to go in and have it completed. What I found very pleasing was when a nurse came over to us and stated there was a bit of a delay due to shortage of equipment and processing of sterilization. I appreciated that so much. She was upfront and honest.

He called me a day later. I went to this local chapel with rosary beads, and I just kept praying.

His voice was very calm and kind. He confirmed what I had and that it was, and I will always remember his statement, "Mrs. Murawski, it is a mere bump in the road."

I needed to hear that because I had a whirlwind of a journey. I kept him as my GI doctor, and once I had a little issue that he helped take right out of commission. I thought he was brilliant. He referred me to another attending physician, who was also two hours away at the same hospital. I went home and within that same week, I had an appointment to see him. The hospital is a 906-bed modern facility in Newark, Delaware. The hospital provides a high level of care only in large scaled teaching hospitals. His office was in an adjacent building right on the main campus of the hospital.

This doctor is a surgical oncologist specialist who has practiced more than thirteen years. He is tall, very slender, athletic, in his early forties, with dark brown hair and a trim beard. He wore casual clothes when I first met him with a lab coat over his attire. He looked at my results and he sat down and explained what he needed to do to remedy the situation.

He said, "There is a small tumor right where your small intestine meets the pancreas, you have a GIST tumor."

I was listening very carefully to his every word.

He said, "It is very small, but it is in the location of the tumor that makes it a bit more involved."

I told him, "I am an operating room nurse."

He said, "You need a Whipple resection."

"A Whipple procedure also known as a pancreatic duodenectomy is an extraordinarily complex operation to remove the head of the pancreas, the first part of the small intestine (duodenum), the gallbladder and the bile duct. The procedure is used to treat tumors and other disorders of the pancreas, intestine and the bile duct. After performing the Whipple resection, the surgeon reconnects the remaining organs to allow you to digest food normally after surgery (Mayo Clinic). The classic Whipple procedure was named after Dr. Allen Whipple, a Columbia University surgeon. It is normal to lose up to 5–10 percent of your body weight after the surgery." (www.webmed.com)

"Because the Whipple resection continues to be one of the most demanding and risky operations for surgeons and patients, the American Cancer society states "it is best to have the procedure done at a hospital that performs at least 15–20 surgeries of this type per year.

What I had was a GIST, which is a gastrointestinal stromal tumor. Gastrointestinal stromal tumors (GISTs) are uncommon cancers that start in special cells in the wall of the gastrointestinal (GI) tract, also known as the digestive tract. The GI tract processes food for energy and rids the body of solid waste. After food is chewed and swallowed, it goes through the esophagus, a tube that carries food down the throat and chest to the stomach. The esophagus joins the stomach just beneath the diaphragm (the thin band of muscle below the lungs).

The stomach is a sac-like organ that helps the digestive process by mixing the food with gastric juices. The food and gastric juices are then emptied into the small intestine. The small intestine, which is about 20 feet long, continues breaking down the food and absorbs most of the nutrients into the bloodstream.

The small intestine joins the large intestine, the first part of which is the colon, a muscular tube about 5 feet long. The colon absorbs water and mineral nutrients from the remaining food matter. The waste left after this process (stool) goes into the rectum, where it is stored until it passes out of the body through the anus.

A Miracle to Save My Life

THE AMERICAN CANCER SOCIETY MEDICAL AND EDITORIAL CONTENT TEAM

"Our team is made up of doctors and oncology certified nurses with deep knowledge of cancer care as well as journalists, editors, and translators with extensive experience in medical writing."

As I WALKED INTO THE ROOM all I could think of was, "Oh my goodness, this is unbelievably incredible." I only remember seeing these in the operating room when patients were given last resort for survival. The doctor said immediately, "You need to have it done."

I began to listen intently to his reasoning.

Then as I sat there, he said, "I have plans to proceed with the surgery in a couple of months after they removed the huge sac near your ovary."

I instantly disagreed with him and said,

"No. You see doctor, I have been through surgery and back before, and you are doing both together."

He shot a surprised look at me as I continued, "I am an extraordinarily strong person. I want this done on the same day.

"Are you sure?" he asked.

"Absolutely." I said with conviction. "Please speak with the gynecology specialist."

The doctor said, "You are strong because you are a nurse"

It was a day or two later the office called. I picked up my phone and a voice on the other end said,

"Mrs. Murawski, your surgery will be done in six weeks."

I was not thrilled with the idea of having to wait so many weeks for them to pursue this incredible feat. But I knew that both specialists would have to concur about the surgery and have the operating room and their operating teams available the same day for this massive surgery. I tried my best not to Google anything on the internet. This could have led me to more problems or concerns, so I stayed away, and I was proud of myself for finding the courage not to explore. I know, I know what anyone reading this must be thinking she is a nurse why isn't she researching and getting herself mentally and physically ready for this? To be honest to myself and anyone else, I had to be real with myself, as a nurse after practicing for over 30 years. I knew the jargon, the drill, and all the procedures by now. If I had the confidence in me to believe that my doctors would take me from my darkest and scariest moments, and I was into a peaceful end, knowing that I will be okay—then it was time to start mentally preparing and to find the solace in that.

Now I began the countdown to the days before the surgery. That part of the process is nerve-wracking in every way. Time seemed to be moving in slow motion. My pain only increased, and my thought processes at times were running out of control. I prayed and prayed and spoke to different people who tried so hard to encourage me and make me hopeful. The one consolation was that it was me, and not my children, who would have to endure this huge obstacle that waited before me.

I went to the beach a few times and walked near the water and stared at the ocean. One time I went with my daughter and we laughed and cried. I felt the beach brought energy to endure what was ahead of me. I felt the sun refueled me in some way. It energized me.

Have Faith—
Believe in Yourself

YOU TRULY MUST BELIEVE in yourself. I am Catholic and I prayed constantly to God. I have prayed so much, read the book of miracles, and listened to *Verses of Healing* online, that a friend once sent me. I have asked God numerous times to just take the pain away. I would also ask to make me normal again. It is not always when we want the healing, but it is on His time.

Therefore, please be patient, rest and heal. It is not at all easy to do when you are in pain, suffering, tired and just plain exhausted, but you must find a way to gather strength and the willpower to beat it. I promise you have it in you.

I had suffered for about a year from onset of pain and have had extensive and scary events as a patient. I even had surgeries years before, major surgery and had minor surgeries as a child. We cannot change our lives.

My mom would always say, and I repeat the line, "It is what it is."

We have to accept the challenges we are given. We must try to do the best that we can to overcome the hurdles in our own way.

I understood first-hand how difficult, frustrating, and sometime hopeless you feel. Today, as I did in the past, I try to be upbeat and enjoy bike riding or just sitting by a pool or spending time with family. We must enjoy and be appreciative for everything we are given. Life is a true gift for all of us.

By my standards, nothing in life is more meaningful than health, love, and family. Health is a priceless gift!

I will never forget these famous words from one of my other sisters. I am the oldest sibling of five. I have three other sisters, and a brother.

She said, "You are in it to win it!"

I kept repeating that to myself time and time again. It was so inspirational to hear that. I am sure to pass that little but valuable phrase on to someone who needs to hear it eventually. It truly helped me.

Let the tears flow, and I mean flow. I never cried so much and as easily as I have in the past year. It is a great release; cleanses the body it makes you feel better and lighter. It seems to remove a load from your heart and shoulders.

I do realize as we get older, it does take more time for us to heal. It is a much slower process. Sometimes two ailments act up together. You are not dealing with one, but may have two or more. It can be overwhelming for sure.

I cannot say this enough, not everyone will experience this in their lives, and I do respect that. I am truly, truly blessed and forever grateful to my loving beautiful husband, Don for helping me even when he was tired, and sick of me, etc. He is not in the medical field. He would drive back and forth two hours each way when I was hospitalized, and when I needed to see the doctors for follow up visits. He was always on my front line to assist and help me in any way. He gave me incredibly good back massages because I carry much of my stress in my lower back. It is awfully hard to see a loved one suffer, and I was on the other end of that too. It is painful to witness. You feel helpless for them and want to help. I will never forget

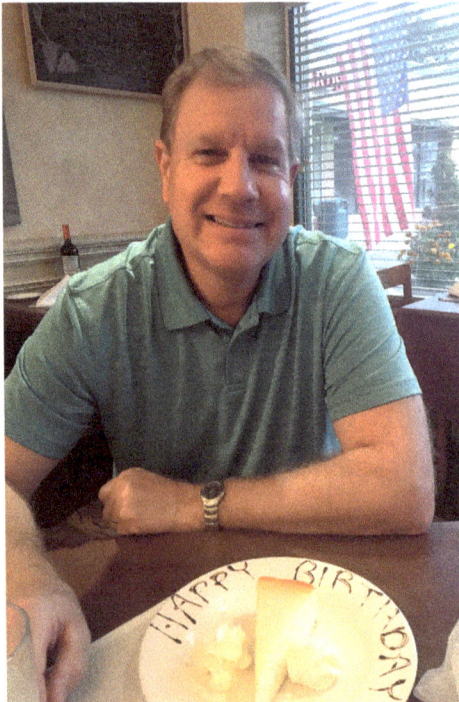

MY incredible husband.

how many times he repeated the process of getting me medications, running to the store for items, checking the internet for information and sometimes getting plain and simply frustrated too. I was not always the best patient and I hate to admit, I am quite stubborn.

With that all said, I am again thankful to my family for the calls, visits, texts, goodies, gifts, well wishes, numerous prayers, religious gifts cards and baskets etc. Without them, I would have been far behind with my healing. I am so happy for the support they provided for me. It gave me more courage and kept me in check. I felt so bad when I cried to my mom at times. I did not want her to ever think I was weak, but I had to vent, and get off my chest the emotional toll I was undergoing. I understand fully when it is your child and they are suffering. It is so hard for a parent to witness a child suffering.

When I went for follow up visits, I was referred to one medical oncologist because they thought I would have to take this target (not chemo) pill for the tumor I had removed to prevent re-occurrence. I made the appointment and again like a walking trooper, I tried to keep it together.

My surgeries were in the past. When I was greeted by a stocky, short, male attending physician, I hoped for the best. He went through all my tests surgeries and said, and I remember those most beautiful words, "Mrs. Murawski, you will not have to take anti-target pills."

I had been anticipating this for a while, and hoped he would say I did not need these pills which also caused many side effects. I asked him to repeat what he said, and I got up and hugged him. My husband and I were so elated. It was very much needed superb news! I felt my smile crease my face and knew that I lit up the world. I was beyond grateful to hear this news.

Revelation of Pregnancy and Parenthood

What Being a Baby Nurse and Mom Truly Means to Me

FOR SOME OF US, it is easy to get pregnant but for others, it is a trying experience in many ways. Month after month of hopes and then letdowns can occur. You either get your period or you miscarry which is devastating, especially when you want a family.

I was working in the operating room at the time, and I asked my doctor, who was also a colleague of mine point blank for a script for Clomid. She was a jovial, attractive doctor who had the best smile I had ever seen.

She said, "I will fill it for you, but you can possibly have twins." She gave the prescription to me right then and there to try without having to see her in her office for a script.

Clomid is an oral prescription that is used to stimulate ovulation. For every 20 pregnancies with clomid, only one results with twins according to statistics.

Clomid can be prescribed by your primary physician, which I frankly did not know. It can also be prescribed by your obstetrical doctor. They usually order this before referring you to a fertility physician, a reproductive endocrinologist who practices a sub-specialty of obstetrics and gynecology which addresses hormonal functioning as it pertains to reproduction and infertility in both men and women.

A pregnancy usually lasts 280 days or 40 weeks' gestation. It is this wonderful elating news that you are pregnant and expecting a bundle of joy! When your pregnancy is confirmed there is this

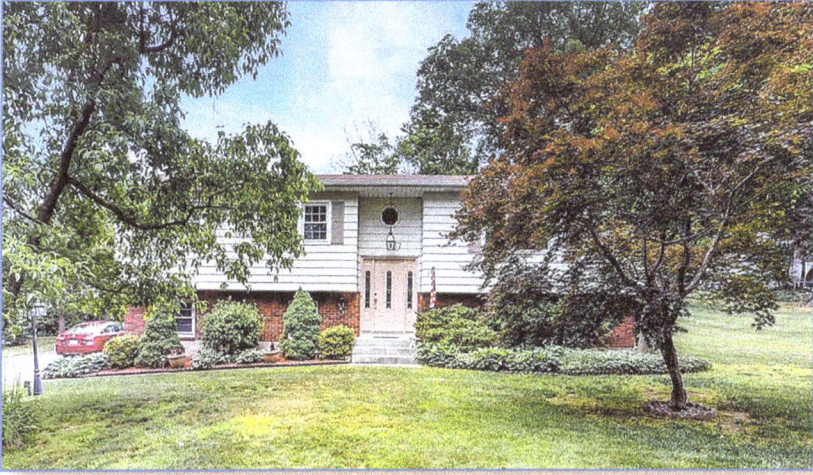

Sweet memories were made in our former house in Rockland County, upstate NY

feeling of unbelief at first, then once you have realized that there is a wee one growing inside of you, your heart beats with joy. This breathtaking news is priceless for both parents-to-be, especially when you really want to have a child of your very own.

It is truly a magical time for both of you. I waited a while to have a child. The timing was great. We moved from a one-bedroom cooperative apartment in Queens, New York to a house in upstate New York called New City, in Rockland County. We traveled, worked hard and saved as best as we could. When I found out, I was shocked quite frankly at the pregnancy urine test, and I kept staring at it. I had bought a rattle a few years prior and waited for that opportune time to tell my husband. I put the test and rattle in a plastic bag and said, "Look under your pillow." The look of pure joy that my husband gave to me will be forever etched in my mind.

Even though I was pregnant I knew enough to be careful as we were going skiing with my two brothers-in-law and their wives. My immediate family was overjoyed and shared in this exciting time in our lives. It had been seven years since we were married. They never asked us about children before that. I had a great trip, and I immediately scheduled an appointment with my obstetrical physician.

After she examined me, she said, "Oh yes, you are pregnant!"

Oh, my goodness, after having the pregnancy confirmed by her, I was just thrilled that I was going to be a mom. I knew right away as my maternal instincts kicked right in that I was having a boy. My husband really thought it was a girl. We had repeated sonograms due to my age at the time, which was 32. The doctor asked us one week if we wanted to know. We both wanted to be surprised but on the other hand, we wanted to be prepared and organized, for example, for the nursery and what to buy as far as clothes, etc.

The technician said, "I see a ball and a bat there and she gave us the picture."

Well mama was right on; we were having a boy! What a glorious day it was!

Then she also said, "Mom, dad, everything looks normal."

Which of course was an enormous relief. We all may want a boy or a girl but in the real world, the health of the baby is of utmost importance.

As time passed during the pregnancy, we attended Lamaze classes for the impending birth. "The goal of Lamaze is to build a mother's confidence in her ability to give birth through the presentation of classes that help prepare women to understand and how to cope with pain in ways that both facilitate labor and to promote comfort including relaxation techniques, movement and massage." (Wikipedia-wiki-Lamaze technique)

In the Lamaze class, we met many couples who like us, were friendly, and who were sharing the joy of being pregnant together. There was one couple who we eventually met up with a few years later. By then our children were toddlers, and we had invited them to our home for dinner.

As the boys grew up, they were in the same elementary classes and worked their way to middle school together. It was very heartwarming to share in this unique connection.

Even as a professional, you really are unaware of the outcome of the birth. Some women have vaginal deliveries, and some have

Cesarean Sections (C-Section). A Cesarean Section is a procedure done in the operating room, involving an incision that is either bilateral, or across the pelvis line, to retrieve the newborn. A C-Section is done sometimes because the babies are too big, not in the right position, are breech, and or is done after long labors that can be devastating and can cause death to the mother and the unborn child. Whichever way you have a baby, the outcome is the same. You are now parents!

I had awfully long labors with both of my children, but I was lucky to have had vaginal deliveries with both. I also received epidurals with both as requested. An epidural is a procedure in which a small catheter is placed in the small of your back, and an anesthesia drug such as an epidural analgesic is injected into the epidural site in your back, to localize the area and take the edge off severe labor. You can opt for a birth plan as discussed with your physician. The plan will be respected throughout your labor, but if complications arise during the delivery process, your labor nurse, and obstetrical staff will do what is needed to do in the best interest of you and your baby. It could be your wish to have the lights low, who you want in labor with you, if you want medications.

My experience as nurse was not in labor or delivery, except for two incidences where I worked with a midwife on two separate birth cases where the nurses were busy. A midwife had asked me to help her deliver a relatively low risk pregnancy. I told her I would, but I just asked her to tell me what she wanted me to do. I followed her lead and did what she told me to do. It just so happens that this happened on two consecutive Fridays. Thank the Dear Lord, all went well with the deliveries.

The patient delivered without any analgesics. It was the second pregnancy for both women. I was also grateful I did not get kicked because I had to watch for a leg that was appearing in my direction during one of those deliveries. I was trying to keep the patient's leg flexed, but she seemed to extend it in my direction after a long painful contraction. I was glad I was paying attention and have decent reflexes.

My specialty was postpartum as I worked with the moms and their babies. I utterly understood all that they were experiencing both as a patient and as a nurse. It is good when you can really empathize with them.

When it came close to having my baby-to-be, I instructed my husband on my plans for labor. As much as I enjoyed the Lamaze classes, I knew as a professional that you do not get a medal for being a hero in the delivery room. Your prize is the healthy baby you carried.

In my birthing plan I specified that I would like medication to take the edge off the labor pain and contractions and make it easier for the transition of birth. My doctor and my husband respected my wishes and quite frankly just wanted everything to be as smooth as possible. I wanted an epidural as soon as I was able to have it.

The anesthesiologist does this procedure for the patient as needed and ordered and requested. I do absolutely respect those patients who want to have a baby naturally. Both of my children took their sweet time to come out. Honestly after a while I wondered if they really wanted to see what the world was like, or what mommy and daddy looked like.

Alas, I endured 22–23 hours with both. I did not think I would have enough strength, but never underestimate to power of a woman, especially a mother.

"I am woman, hear me roar" is a lyric from 'I Am Woman', by Helen Reddy (1971). It is a beautiful song that tells of the strength of women. Attributing other women in their strength to be a woman in a world where women even today are often expected to be submissive. But not us—when it comes to our children, lyrics from Katy Perry's song 'Roar' come to-mind: "I got the eye of the tiger, a fighter, dancing through the fire, 'cause I am a champion and you're gonna hear me roar, louder, louder than a lion."

I find this most like women when they are in labor. We women are like a Tigress or Lioness protecting her babe while she is giving them up from her own body into the world.

Once you have a baby, and even if the labor is long—Once the baby is cleaned up and placed in your arms, you may be utterly exhausted but have an undeniable energy and overwhelming feeling of love. Your precious baby is here, and you did it!

Now the reality starts to set in once you have reached your capacity, the adrenalin from your labor and delivery drops significantly. You feel like a truck ripped you open and all you want to do is sleep. Hormones are all over the board in your body, you have just endured a birth and many emotions are running rampant. Visitors are coming or calling. The baby or babies if you had multiples are due to eat. You have cramps and now have your vaginal bleeding back with you, but it's not the period you get every month it's much worse as you have all this blood and uterine lining to expel from your body. You may be quite hungry as you could not eat for the whole of your labor and were just given ice chips to moisten your mouth, and then again you are just plain out tired and do not want to eat at all. In the post-partum room the nurse will continue to give you IV fluids and maybe a pain-killer and help you with nursing the baby if that is what you choose.

You are trying your best to make it all right in the world and for your new bundle. As a mother and a nurse, I totally get it in every way. Visitors are a nice surprise and make the birth of your child a joyful event, but sometimes they stay—and—do not—leave!

When this happened, I hated to do this, but I really wanted time with my baby and my husband—alone. I had to whisper in my husband's ears to ask him to please tell his parents that they needed to leave as they were endlessly staying in the room.

I had to use the bathroom. Women know who have been through labor and delivery, it takes us longer than the normal than usual time to go to the bathroom. You are bleeding, you are shedding clots, and you need to clean up and put a clean pad on. It hurts and you are uncomfortable. Not only does it hurt, but you may have had to have an episiotomy which is a surgical cut made at the opening of the vagina during childbirth, to aid a difficult delivery and prevent rupture of tissues. It can make you feel quite sore until you are fully healed. (https://www.mayoclinic.org/healthy-lifestyle/labor-and-delivery/in-depth/episiotomy/art-20047282)

Besides our post-partum functions, we must try to begin nursing our newborn, or choose bottle-feeding. Nursing a newborn can be quite tedious for both the mom and baby.

As a post-partum nurse, I would summon the husband and say your wife looks tired. If they were not married, I would just say mom looks tired. Please ask the visitors to leave soon. I understood this from both sides of the bed, the reality of parenthood.

When I had my son, I chose to try to breastfeed him, but I found it a challenge. I was patient with myself, but I found that my son was always hungry. Although you want to breast feed, you are tired and having your child on you to feed, is at times relentless, even though you know it is for the good of both of you.

One incentive for the mom is that you do lose weight when nursing, but you must keep your calories up to provide yourself and baby with good nutrition. You must also drink plenty of water, so you do not get dehydrated and constipated. Frankly, I did not drink enough. For the baby it is great because baby gets all your antibodies help them grow well and healthy those first few months of their precious lives.

Many mothers feel the urge to nurse, as it is better for both mom and baby. But at times this may not be feasible, if it is not your full intention, due to either pressure from others, or just from feeling uncomfortable with the whole idea. Bottle-feeding is fine too. Don't feel guilty over your decision at all whether to nurse or bottle-feed.

Nowadays, there are breastfeeding consultants called Lactation Counselors, who are great at what they do. I have had the pleasure of working with them and I think they rock! As a patient, I did not have those fine individuals around at the time. I am not sure the hospital utilized them, or they did not have that specific role.

It is a most wonderful time, one to enjoy always, remembering and looking back with smiles. It was tiresome but all worth it, and as one friend of mine once said, "They grow up fast."

It is so, so true.

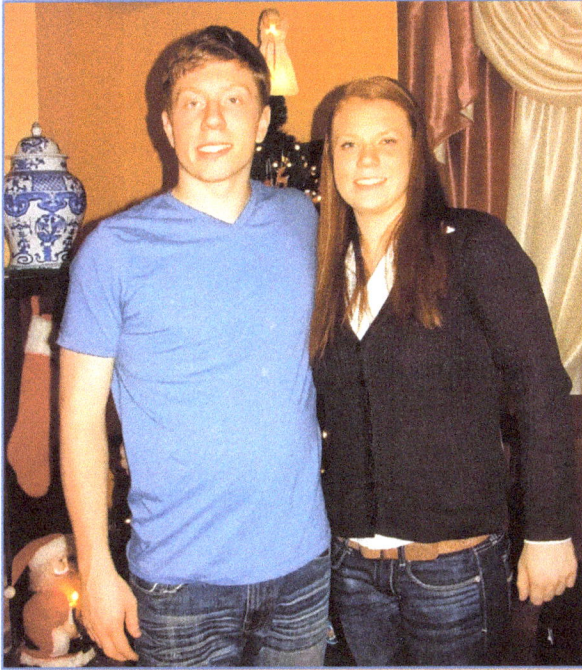

Two close siblings. (I took this picture in our house in upstate New York.)

Baby Number Two— My Daughter Jillian

WHEN I WAS EXPECTING my second child, I had a toddler who was full of endless energy. Ryan Patrick Murawski gave us a run for our time, with initials RPM, which means 'rotations per minute' or revolutions per minute. I wanted him to have my dad's name as his middle name.

Ryan was so much fun. He was a happy child, but full of energizer batteries. For those who have raised that 'on the go' toddler while caring for a newborn baby, you know what it is like to try and keep an eye on them, and make sure your baby is cared for at the same time. If your older child is still in diapers and needs potty training, that is a whole other ball game, which is like 'keeping up with the Jones.'

Nobody questioned me, and if they did, I would have told them my motives and reasons. Mothers, what we feel is normal for ourselves is truly our truth for rearing our children. I feel this way. I saw women in post-partum chose to bottle-feed their newborn. They had their reasons and I saw the joy on their faces as they fed that babe whether it was with the breast or the bottle. What matters is that the baby is being nourished, cared for and loved—that is how the bond forms, and that is all that matters.

I was bottle-fed and I feel I am fine. I truly did not want that guilt factor in any way to be an issue about not nursing my daughter Jillian, and it was through the experiences of the mothers in the nursery that I was able to learn so much.

Jillian was such an easygoing baby and toddler. She slept well too. I was so grateful because Ryan was a poor sleeper. Yep, like I said, he was my RPM day and night. One wonders how I kept up. But mothers do. It is in our genetics.

Time Has a Way
of Passing Us By

A S THE YEARS FLEW BY, my children grew up fast. I wanted to do something in nursing that gave me so much joy. My nurse manager asked me if I wanted to teach classes for mothers and fathers to be. I was so happy to be given the opportunity and decided that it was a great way to help parents in the journey of their new lives as parents.

I searched out information and went to classes that nurses in the post-birthing units were giving. I was deep down thrilled to train for this new moment in my nursing career. Now as a mother and a nurse, I could explain and teach them some helpful tips to take home to make the transition so much easier.

My children were the first on both sides of the family. I admit that although as I grew up, I watched my parents raise their kids, they were both loving and caring. But now it was my turn and being the oldest of five I did not have a sibling who had children to show me what it was like to be a parent. For me being a mom at times felt alienating because I was the first to have children of my own. Nowadays, I just want love and respect as a parent too.

So, I put my nurse's cap on and tried to apply taking care of my children as what I saw my mother do, what I watched in the nursing room of the hospital, and through my own trials and errors.

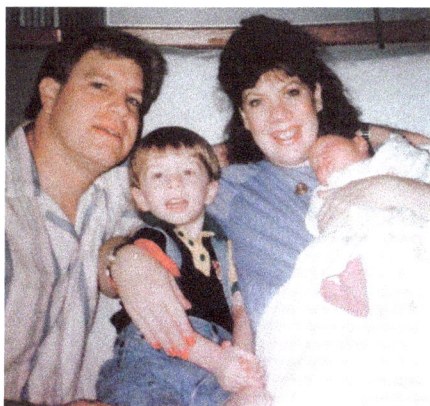

Family is priceless and forever cherished. A nurse took this picture in the hospital where Jill was delivered in Rockland County, NY

I always said, as a parent, but especially as a mom, kids will never know unless you tell them. You do not have to tell them what you did wrong. You are not being graded or judged. Don't put so much pressure on yourself. We are not perfect and just try our best. This is what I conveyed to my new parents.

Once I researched my information, did some reading, watched other classes, and started what would eventually become a lifelong full passion teaching Mother and Baby Classes.

I have been a nurse since I graduated from nursing school in 1984, through 2018. I really thought I enjoyed the specialties that I learned along the way. I was ready to take on the new experience that I would be able to teach from both sides of the bed. The first hospital was in Westchester in Tarrytown, NY. I liked to teach but really did not get the most passion out of it until I went to Greenwich, Connecticut and my good friend and manager approached me with the idea. I grabbed it quickly. I worked postpartum with moms and taught the mother baby classes. It was fun to see the patients who I taught find comfort and patience in becoming a new mom and bonding with their baby.

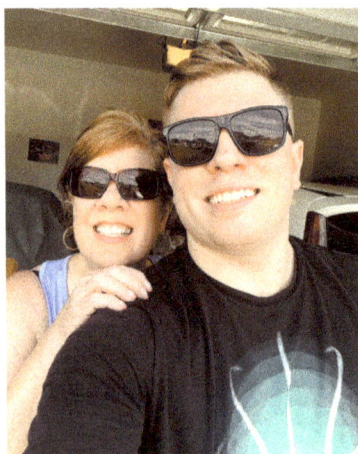

My Ryan

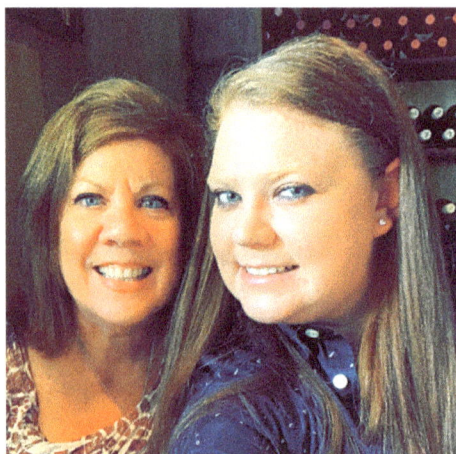

My Jilly

Baby Care Classes and Instruction

FOR THIS NURSE to be able to teach these new parents, I felt it was vital for me to come up with a care plan. I typed up a brief baby care format that I thought was important to the learning needs of my patients. I kept revising it, adding and deleting information along the way to keep up with the trends of modern parenting and nurturing. It was the most endearing to me to see the attentiveness of the parents-to-be. My instructional was a two-hour class. The first hour was learning guides and tips; the second hour was hands on bathing, diapering, and handling of dolls.

The class was held in a long conference room with cozy chairs, and I made sure the room was cool enough to keep them awake. They brought their food and drink and I tried to make it as informal as I could. The cherry table in the room held a folder containing information not covered in class, and additional tips to take home, or read at their convenience. It was also functional to be able to practice baby changing and so on. Below, I will explain what I think is crucial to know and keep in the back of your mind.

Nurse Georgia's Baby Care Plan

MAKE SURE BEFORE THE BABY ARRIVES, you make an appointment with a pediatrician, one who has been recommended by either your obstetrician, the hospital, or someone you know who trusts this doctor. You want to become familiar with the office and make sure they accept your insurance. Write down any questions you may have for the pediatrician. The nursery staff provides you with a chart with all the baby information, from the time they are born until they are discharged from the hospital to give to the pediatrician's office.

If you have a baby shower, here are a few suggestions for easy and inexpensive items to put in your 'party registration package.' A Safety Kit, with a rectal thermometer, pacifiers, a two-in-one purpose playpen that can be used as a sleeper and playpen, gates when they are mobile. If you are purchasing anything that has been used, such as car seats and strollers, make sure there are no recalls. A car seat is mandatory and vital for the child's safety in the car. If there is a flaw it can cause death to a child. Police stations can help with testing and assisting you with car seats. Some strollers look great, but had mechanisms that were faulty. This has caused children to be folded into the carriage while the mother is pushing it.

These are mandatory items and concerns young parents must think about before their baby is in enters the world.

You must have baby clothes you can wash. You should keep some items that are in larger sizes. Infants can grow out of the newborn (0–3 months) sizes quickly especially if you had a big baby, which is considered about eight pounds or over at birth.

Do not use too much detergent. I used Dreft laundry detergent and I think used too much. Today there are many choices and varieties, including Seventh Generation, and Puracy Natural liquid detergent). You may want to use detergents that are free of dyes or fragrances.

Make sure you have a support person, whether it is your husband, boyfriend, mom, best friend, sister to really help you during this time. He/she can cook, clean, wash clothes, run errands, or help feed the baby with prepared food.

Familiarize yourself with new gadgets or items you will use for your baby. Make sure you know how to use the car seat before bringing your infant home; practice placing it in the bracket in the car, and removing it. I remember one time when I wheeled down my patient for discharge, the father was sweating and struggling with the base of the seat. I felt so bad for him. We are not required to have to show the parent how to use the seats, but I tried to assist him.

When traveling in a vehicle, the baby should be in the rear, and be rear-facing.

The Boppy pillow, which is used for positioning a baby for breast-feeding, is a good purchase. It is a U-shaped soft pillow for the newborn to lay on while breastfeeding. Please bring it to hospital, but keep it in the original case or put it in a pillowcase. This will help keep the pillow clean and free of germs.

Pets and the New Baby

IF YOU HAVE A PET OR PETS, please bring a hat home that the baby had on his or her head. The animal or animals can get to smell the newborn's scent before he/she comes home. When you do come home, have one parent give the animal attention and one give attention to the baby. It is new for everyone. Do not leave the baby unattended. No matter how nice your pet is, it needs to get adjusted to the new family member and will be curious. Do not ignore your pet, and make sure the animal's nails are short. Animals get jealous too and we must be vigilant to watch how they are around the baby. No matter how well you know your pet, they are animals.

Special Visitors for Our New Baby

WHEN VISITING FAMILY OR FRIENDS, please keep the car seat at your height and not on the floor. Small children other pets or you could accidentally kick the car seat while not knowing it. By having it at your height and next to you, you are being more of a protective mother bear, so to speak, and it tells everyone in the room that this child is now a part of the family and should be respected as such.

Skin-to-skin contact is totally beneficial for bonding. The uterus was the baby's first home and once born, there is a lot of stimulus around, and it can be overwhelming. The closeness of skin-to-skin contact is important for maintaining blood sugar, calming baby, and keeping heart rate down and soothing fussiness. Talk or sing (or both) to the baby since she/he knows your voice from being inside of you. Dads can do skin to skin as well by holding their new bundle on their naked chest with a blanket on top of them creating a nurturing safe place that is both calming and loving for the newborn. It helps new dads bond with their child in the way moms bond with the child while nursing.

I remember one instance when I was working, and I heard a baby crying. I quickly walked up the hallway and noted it was one of my patients. I went into the mom's room and she had the baby in the baby Isolette. An Isolette is a clear plastic enclosed crib maintaining a warm environment and helps the baby isolate from other germs. I instantly jumped into action but in a calm quiet way. The first-time mother was crying and did not know what to do. I immediately washed my hands and gently took the baby out of the Isolette.

The new mom looked so devastated, and I could see she did not know what to do. "Mom, I am here to help." Her tears said everything and all she could do was say, "What can I do?"

"Mommy, everything is going to be okay. Here, open your gown and lay the baby vertical on your chest, keep him warm, and start singing or talking to him.

She was sobbing, "What should I say?" As I lay the baby down on her I could feel how shaky she was. Part of the reason is that our hormones raging all over us after we give birth. As I laid the baby down on her, I smiled and gave her a tissue to wipe her tears.

Then I said, "Mom just calm your voice as though you are whispering and say whatever you want to your son." She wiped her face and then took her son so gently under her robe and began talking to him.

"Hi Honey," I heard her say, "Mommy loves you so much."

The baby stared at his mother and the mom stared back. I instantly welled up with tears at this wonderous gesture of love I witnessed. She continued, and I explained to her to tell him what his nursery looked like and what his name would be.

In what seemed like a few moments, he stopped his crying. I touched the mom and simply said,

"Great job!" She looked up at me and gave me this big smile of relief. Then I suggested, "I am just down the hall at the nurses' station, if you need me; I am here for you."

As I walked out of the room, I heard her saying again and again, "Your mommy loves you so much."

We all need encouragement even if it is a small gesture or praise. We need it most when we are most vulnerable. It makes a big difference in our lives and goes a long way.

If the baby's nails are sharp, do not cut them like I did as a first-time parent. Please use a nail file, as it is safer. As they have tiny fingers, use a small nail file if possible. It is hard to figure out if they are crying because they are hungry, tired, bored, wet, or cold. You will be able to identify the cries after a little while.

Stay attuned to the clues.

SIDS: A Killer Among Newborns

CCORDING TO AMERICAN Association of Pediatrics (AAOP) Sudden Infant Death Syndrome (SIDS) has been reduced for babies with safe sleep on their backs. I know this is not the way our parents put us to sleep in the old days which was on our tummy. Babies have been known to drown or choke to death on their own vomit or saliva. Placing them on their back helps them to breathe better.

Keep the bassinette or crib clear and free for baby to move and toss and turn. Do not keep extra toys or thick blankets inside with your newborn. Crib bumpers are not recommended by AAOP, as babies can roll under them and smother or be strangled by fastening laces.

A few other beneficial tips are to make sure you wash your hands frequently, and cover your face if you have a cold. The house temperature should be 68–72° with an average of 70°. Natural light is good. Avoid drafts from windows and air conditions. Babies are fine to sleep in the room with mom, but not advised to sleep in the bed with parents to prevent suffocation. I say this wisely, as parents who are sleeping in the same bed as the baby can easily roll on top of their sleeping baby without knowing, and crush the child or stifle the child to death.

My strong suggestion is to use a bassinette for as long as the baby can sleep in it—once the baby grows you will need to go straight to a crib, until it is time for their first toddler bed.

Practice safe habits from the start.

I am very much into infant safety. Make sure you have a first aid kit and a rectal thermometer in the house because if the baby is sick and they develop a fever, take the temperature right from the start. Make sure you have Vaseline to put on the tip of the thermometer before you penetrate the child's rectum. Keep these two items together by the baby's changing table, this way so you never have to look for it.

A digital one thermometer is fine and the one across the forehead version provides quick notification, but for a better gauge of how high the temperature is, you want to use the rectal temperature as protocol, and accuracy for what may be ailing your baby. Have the pediatrician's phone number in your phone and on the fridge. Also write down the temperature you get when the temperature is taken.

If you think the baby looks ill, acts lethargic, does not eat or drink, or has diarrhea or constipation, there is always a doctor available to belay any fears. The pediatrician's office will ask you almost immediately what the baby's temperature is. When babies are sick and have high temperatures at times they cry so much because they do not feel well and cannot tell you what is wrong. This is normal.

You are probably overwhelmed at this point, so before you call your pediatrician, put your baby safely down in the crib, then you can focus on your call. This way you can tell them what is wrong, and they will evaluate whether you need to make an appointment. It is good practice to write down when the baby ate last, so you can possibly see a pattern, and just be aware of the time when they last ate. Some infants are allergic to formulas that can make them extremely sick, and can cause a high temperature. This is the reason why writing their menu down is important.

Once you and baby are home again, after you have given him medication (if he needs one) and feed him, try to sleep when the baby does. You need to get refueled to be able to take care of both of you. Let the errands or chores in the house alone. Your baby is your priority.

Remember, some babies eat every 2.5 hours, some 3, some 4 hours. Always hold their heads initially because they do not have strength to do it. So please remember to do this. Remember portable gates for stairs when they become mobile. Put plastic plug covers in outlets to prevent unnecessary finger injuries from curiosity. You can pick them up in your local hardware store.

Children love to put things in their mouths. You may need cabinet locks and toilet seat locks too. My son loved to put miniature cars in the toilet water (yikes) ... you don't want those going down the drain and clogging your toilet—No you do not!!

It is my wish here that the information I have provided for you is most important for parenthood. Most of the material has been initiated from the American Association of Pediatrics and my training as a nurse.

As for me, I only wanted my kids to be safe, healthy, and happy in life and as a nurse I want to make sure that other children have the same. If I have those three basic elements, I can give them to other parents. Not only does it make me a content mom, but a gratified nurse, that through the years I did my job well.

As my children grew and matured to be their own persons, I just love to physically see them. To me it gave me the greatest joy in my heart when I can look at them, converse with them, kiss or hug them. I have told them this, so they know how I feel and when they give me that look, you know the look, I mean the one that makes us parents melt.

As a parent now of adults, I know that although they are grown, they still need their parents and I truly know in my heart and soul that they love their mom and their dad very much. That is all this woman needs to go on and be strong in life. My mom still tells me to drink water, keep cool, and wear a sweater or coat when it is cold out. A parent is always a parent, no matter what the age.

Epilogue

THE PURPOSE OF THIS BOOK is to inform you about the many experiences I have endured over the years. I want you to know I am with you, and I totally understand the challenges you may experience. I have had an older neighbor tell me that she never really had surgery ever. It is still important to give and know some information to provide you the best possible outcome. Whether it is a small procedure that is done in the doctor's office under local or general anesthesia, it is still surgery.

I waited patiently for over a year just to learn and play Pickleball. When I got on that court my toughness and competitiveness came out. I was there, physically standing on that court, ready to play a new sport, and my new hobby. Oh yes, the next few days my legs burned and were sore, but I simply did not mind and thought, this is only the beginning of a workout. I had to build up my endurance and stamina once again.

It has been over a year now, and I am looking back a bit, while marching forward and sometimes I just cannot believe what was done to this body. I am enjoying my life to the best of my abilities and I frequently ask people I know who are ailing, "How are you feeling?". I am almost back to myself. I don't have to nap that much anymore, and I enjoy the simple pleasures, like a sunset or the warmth of the sun, or talking to my neighbors and friends about things going on in the community. I like to ask and learn about various topics.

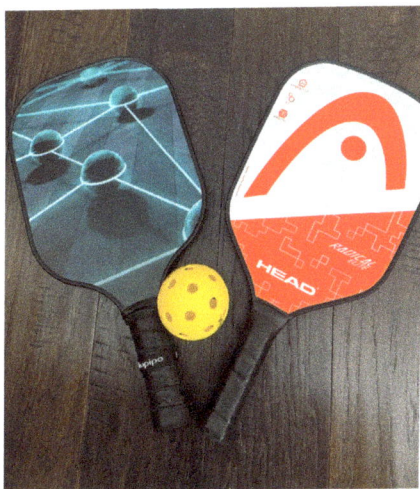

My latest hobby—Pickleball

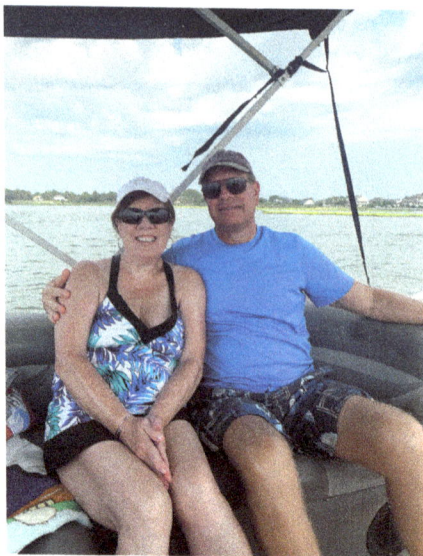

Enjoying simple pleasures of life
— Relaxing

In conclusion, I want to thank you, my readers, for allowing me to inform and enlighten you. I truly and completely understand the hardships, setbacks, and difficult days that you may encounter. I hope I have helped you in some form, and I wish you all the best, now, and in the future.

I am truly thankful to all the doctors, and surgeons who have helped me and saved my life because I was very frightened beyond anyone's knowledge. Overcome as best you can any setbacks big or small you may have along the way. Find joy in the little things that we may otherwise overlook. Just recently I went for a bike ride with my husband in my community, and I held my head high and had a big smile on my face when I was greeted by neighbors. I was so incredibly pleased I could do this, and it gave me a ton of happiness. As I rode my bicycle, I gave them the biggest wave.

I look at my garden and note the beauty in the colors, and the array of growth among the flowers and plants. I look at sunshine and sunsets in a heartwarming way. I look at myself in the mirror and see a happy person who will always be appreciative for the second and third chances I received in life.

I tell people I love them more frequently nowadays; life is so fragile and unpredictable. We must live each day as if it were our last. I tell my best friend, always do one thing for yourself each day. We are all so deserving of this.

My dad would always say life was short. He succumbed to cancer many years ago, and Melanoma was the cause. (It is the deadliest form of skin cancer that travels and spreads).

He taught me both strength and to really appreciate life. I forever talked to him during my rough spots and asked him to help me build more endurance and to give me even more strength. He was one heck of a dad, and I would not trade him for the world even though he died young. I know deep down in my heart, he helped me many times and watched over me.

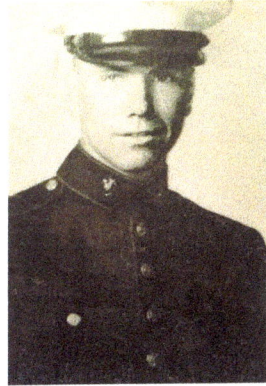

True Warrior—
My dad as a Marine

My sincere advice to everyone who has taken this journey with me; please keep marching forward. Many times, I would say, "I am going to win this battle!"

Sometimes we need to dig deep for extra endurance and determination. We must be vigilant about our bodies and recognize any symptoms that may arise and that are out of the ordinary. If you think something is amiss, please don't let it go, and don't wait. Women wait about thirty-seven minutes longer than men before they contact anyone for medical advice. A delay like this could render a serious outcome. This is according to researchers in Switzerland.

It is a challenge in many ways to withstand pain or anything that is being exhibited. There were times I thought I was in a dream. Reach down for every ounce of strength and willpower because sometimes you may need it. You are strong and you can do this.

One day recently, I wanted to go for a simple bike ride in the neighborhood. However, my bicycle was up on storage hooks in the garage, and nobody was around to help me lift the bike off the hooks that were high on the garage wall. I said a little prayer and asked for undeniable strength. I lifted the bicycle off one of the hooks, and while holding it up I said to myself, "Georgia, you have to get it off the other hook."

Out of the blue, I had this overpowering strength. I lifted the bike up high, and off both hooks.

I held that bike up in the air and placed it on the drive-way and laughed to myself, "Where there is a will, there is a way."

This handy guide is my special gift for you.

May God bless you, now and always!

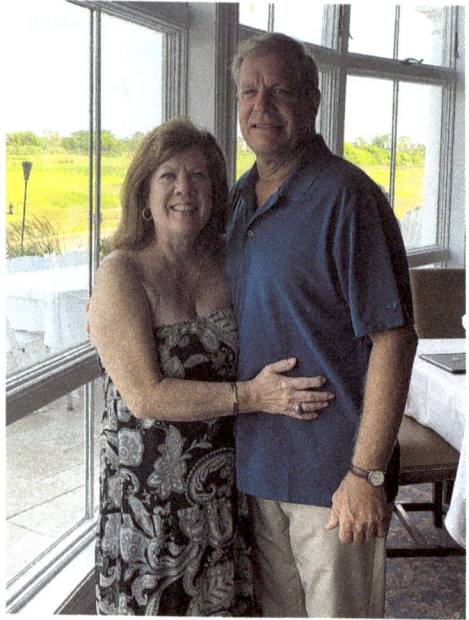

Our 35th wedding anniversary celebration.

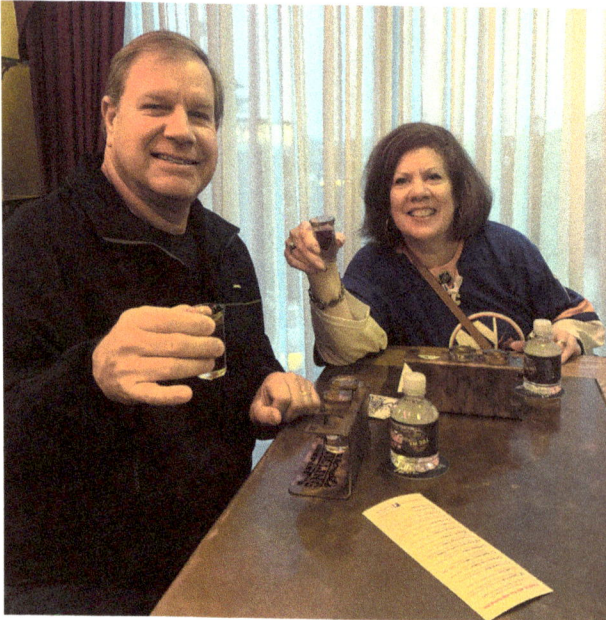

Cheers to Good Health!

BIBLIOGRAPHY

Allina Health Patient Education. *Complete Recovery May take 4–8 hours, 2020.*

American Association of Pediatrics. Moon, Rachel. *How to Keep Your Sleeping Baby Safe: AAP Policy Explained*, December 23, 2020.

American Cancer Society. *Targeted Drug Therapy for Gastrointestinal Stromal Tumors*, May 18, 2020.

American Medical Writer's Association (AMUAA). Turner, Terry. *A hernia is a protrusion of intestinal abdominal fat, 2020.*

Avanos Pain Management. *On Q* Pain Relief System, 2020.*

Cooley, Laura, Senior Director Education and Outreach Academy of Communication in Healthcare. *Fostering Human Connection Covid-19 Virtual Health Care Realm,* May 20, 2020.

European Heart Journal. *Blood pressure medicine more effective when taken at night,* October 27, 2019.

healthline.com. *What is pulse oximetry?* 2020.

hopkinsmedicine.org. *Computerized Tomography (CT),* 2020.

Komen, Susan, Radiology article. *Accuracy of Mammography,* May 5, 2020.

Lamaze International. Hosley Stewart, Darienne. *The Lamaze Method of Childbirth. BabyCenter,* 2007.

Medical News Today. *MRI Scans, Definitions, Uses and Procedure,* July 21, 2018.

Mayo Clinic. *CT Scan,* February 28, 2020.

Mayo Clinic. *Whipple Procedure,* June 3, 2020.

mayoclinic.org/healthy-lifestyle/pregnancy-week-by-week/in-depth/pregnancy/art-20044568. *Childbirth classes: Get ready for labor and delivery,* September 29, 2020.

www.ingramcontent.com/pod-product-compliance
Lightning Source LLC
Chambersburg PA
CBHW041300040426
42334CB00028BA/3107